HEALTH CARE ISSUES, COSTS AND ACCESS

TRANSFUSION - THINK ABOUT IT

HEALTH CARE ISSUES, COSTS AND ACCESS

Additional books in this series can be found on Nova's website under the Series tab.

Additional E-books in this series can be found on Nova's website under the E-books tab.

HEALTH CARE ISSUES, COSTS AND ACCESS

TRANSFUSION - THINK ABOUT IT

TREVOR J. COBAIN
EDITOR

Nova Science Publishers, Inc.
New York

For permission to use material from this book please contact us:
Telephone 631-231-7269; Fax 631-231-8175
Web Site: http://www.novapublishers.com

LIBRARY OF CONGRESS CATALOGING-IN-PUBLICATION DATA

Transfusion : think about it / editor, Trevor J. Cobain.
p. ; cm.
Includes bibliographical references and index.
ISBN 978-1-61668-969-8 (hardcover)
1. Blood--Transfusion. 2. Burns and scalds--Surgery. I. Cobain, Trevor J.
[DNLM: 1. Blood Transfusion. 2. Blood. WB 356 T7746 2010]
RM171.T732 2010
615'.39--dc22
2010025687

Published by Nova Science Publishers, Inc. ✦ New York

CONTENTS

FOREWORD

Burn surgery requires an infrastructure to ensure safe and accurate debridement of the necrotic burnt tissue. Blood products are a vital piece of the jigsaw, to ensure maintenance of a circulating volume and facilitate haemostasis. Is there such thing as a “routine” transfusion? The transfusion needs to be a "tailored” transfusion to meet the specific needs of the individual. Each major burn I have treated has been unique with a unique set of problems to solve. One problem is maintenance of the circulation during surgery. We need to understand how to replace like with like where ever possible. Working collaboratively will give our patients the best possible outcomes. My experiences at the time of the Bali bombing are such an example. We explored the use of fresh whole blood and reduced our transfusion needs with stable clotting profiles. This was achieved by team work, with a clear understanding that a multidisciplinary approach is vital in survival and the quality of the survival.

Fiona Wood, AM. Director of Burn Services of Western Australia working at Royal Perth Hospital and Princess Margaret Hospital for Children. Clinical Professor with the School of Paediatrics and Child Health at the University of Western Australia. Director of the McComb Research Foundation. Australian of the Year 2005.

INTRODUCTION

Trevor J. Cobain

South Eastern Area Laboratory Services (SEALS), South Eastern and Illawarra Area Health Service, Sydney, New South Wales, Australia.

It could be argued that Transfusion is a unique medical event.

It can have outstanding positive outcomes. It is often readily identifiable as a life saving/essential requirement. It can also have some severe negative outcomes but, fortunately these are very rare.

Some of the negative events have been "unknown" or essentially unknown until they have been discovered in those who have received transfusion. This is particularly so with emerging infections and some of the less understood infectious agents.

It is a very highly regulated area and it is a very emotive area.

There are some who are very negative about transfusion. Some of these convictions are based on religious beliefs but some are built on ignorance. A very useful set of data has come from the section of the community who have refused transfusion [1,2].

It is an area of medicine that in many nations relies on altruism to be successful. Although this is the case it is a very expensive part of the health system.

There are areas within the transfusion system that are very difficult to discuss openly. There is some concern when comparing blood product use between hospitals. There is some protection when discussing methods, product quality, costs , risks, availability of products from fractionators – particularly when they are privately owned and are reliant on share price or responsible for delivering a dividend to the share holders.

Quite often we are dealing with products that have extremely demanding storage requirements, with dramatic consequences if these are not met. In addition the shelf life of some of the products is relatively short.

Some of the quality control measures can only be achieved by destructive testing.

Identification for the use of this product is almost unique.

Guidelines, measures of appropriateness, regulations are all useful in identifying when a transfusion should be given but it can be reasonably argued that each transfusion is a unique event.

The choice of product is extremely important. How is this decided? Who decides what products are available? Is it directly related to cost? How do you calculate the "whole of health" cost – particularly the part that is affected by which blood product is used?

The priorities for blood transfusion are not always clear.

There are many competing forces. Not least of which are the priorities of the organizations that are producing the blood products and the organizations who are transfusing the blood products.

All of those involved have some very reasonable interests.

Table 1 endeavors to summarize some of these and how they may (at times) be in conflict.

Table 1

Priority Item	Expected				
	Patient	Clinician	Producer	Donor	Hospital
Product Availability	Yes	Yes			
No Risk	Yes			Yes	Yes
Best Product		Yes			
Freshest Product		Yes			
Following Regulations			Yes		
Stay within Budget			Yes		
Meet production Target			Yes		
No Waste			Yes		Yes
Make a difference				Yes	
Efficient use of product				Yes	
Follow Guidelines					Yes
Cheapest Product					Yes
Eye on Share Price?			Yes		

PRIORITIES OF PRODUCTION

The priorities of Production are numerous and complex:

How can they get the required number and type of donors and at the right time? How do they work out how many they need? What is the best method for making the products that are required? How do they make these products while staying within budget and while satisfying all of the regulatory demands that are often changing [3,4]. Are the priorities of production: a safe product, one that will give large numbers and one that is not expensive? The funding arrangements for many of those charged with the responsibility of producing blood products has been substantially changed over the past 10 years. They have been modified from being an altruistic organization to a business that is answerable to Government for a budget and for a level of production within an extremely stringent set of requirements set down by various regulatory systems. For instance in Australia The Australian Red Cross Blood Service was established in 1996, the Commonwealth Serum Laboratories were privatized in 1994 and the National Blood Authority came into existence on the 1st July 2003.[1]

PRIORITIES OF TRANSFUSION

The priorities of transfusion are frequently indicated by guidelines [5-9], audits [10-12] and measures of appropriateness [13-21]. Often these criteria are almost traditional. The best product is the product that the clinician requires. Or is it? Sometimes the cost of blood products is now apportioned to the hospitals using them. Under these circumstances the cost is clearly a factor. It is not simply a case that the most expensive blood product will lead to an expensive outcome for all patients. Is it possible that expensive blood products can actually decrease costs in other ways (such as length of stay)? Some how there is a requirement to have a very good understanding of "whole of health" cost. There is more and more an expectation that we are heading towards specific products and medicine for a specific patient, and one that will not cost the hospital too much.

In short the transfusionist is looking for the best product for the patient while often the production authority is focused on getting the required number of donors, providing a blood product that will not go out of date before it is used and staying within the budget that has been provided by the funding agency.

In addition and somewhere within this framework there is the Laboratory Blood Bank and the Regulatory Agency. How do they fit into all of this?

The Laboratory Blood Bank has a clear responsibility to negotiate some level of stock with the Production facility and also has the responsibility for crossmatching and identifying red cell and other antibodies or special requirements for each patient. In some instances they may also maintain an antibody register to minimize adverse transfusion outcome. There is some debate as to the role they have or should have in monitoring, advising or enforcing transfusion guidelines and overall blood product usage. It is a very difficult and demanding role. It can be argued that surely the responsibility for blood usage is with the transfusionist (hospital). They are actually administering the blood and it is that institution (in many cases now) that are responsible for the majority of the blood product budget. On the other hand the Laboratory Blood Bank is often the institution that has all the information that identifies how the blood products have been used and also how much has expired or been wasted.

How does the Regulatory agency fit into this? The answer to this is probably that they set the rules and then make sure that they are followed and that the standard of the production and also to some extent the issuing/prescribing facilities are maintained at the required level. This is obviously a huge responsibility as there is a very clear expectation by the community (the recipient of blood products) that there is very little or "no" risk related to having a blood transfusion. There is also an expectation of the blood donor that their donation will be fully utilized and not wasted in any way. The situation is also such that the regulatory institution

---

[1] The National Blood Authority (NBA) is an Australian Government statutory agency, established under the *National Blood Authority Act 2003* to improve and enhance the management of the Australian blood and plasma product sector at a national level. The NBA represents the interests of the Australian, state and territory governments, and sits within the Australian Government's Health and Ageing portfolio.
The NBA is jointly funded by all governments with the National Government contributing 63% and the States 37%.

has the capability to have a very significant impact on blood stocks and also on the type of blood products that are available for transfusion. The licensing of a product can influence the release of that product. The availability of regular products can also be influenced by quarantining product or even more so during a product recall. The balance of all of this can be delicate and there is a huge responsibility to get the correct balance between safety and what could be interpreted as over-regulation [22]. There are a huge number of restrictions and regulations that are imposed today compared to 20 years ago or even 10 years ago. These have had implications for the availability of donors, the speed at which products can be produced, the availability of products and the safety of blood products.

Throughout all of these aspects of transfusion there is a huge revival in the interest of data that is available on all aspects of transfusion as it is extremely difficult to understand any of these issues without complete and accurate data. This in itself is a real challenge as the data may not be readily available and some alternatives are very time consuming.

This data can be huge. Many of the systems that are currently in use may not have the capability to deliver this information in an ideal format. However, there are ways that at least some information can be determined.

Plasma Products

There is one major issue relating to transfusion that is not included in this book. This is relating to plasma products and the future and new products that are currently in production or are "on the drawing board". This area is huge and needs to be left to a more specific group of experts. However, a few suggestions have been provided by one who has been at the forefront of this area for many years.[2]

The future of plasma products and specifically the development of any new products from plasma is a topic which has not been directly addressed in this book. The reason for this is that over the last five to ten years the plasma fractionation industry has undergone a series of significant changes. The not-for-profit national fractionators, largely based in Europe, have either shut down, been bought by commercial fractionators or are seeking amalgamation in the face of intense competition from the small group of large multinational commercial fractionators. Those that remain will have difficulty surviving into the next decade while the large multinational commercial fractionators will continue to consolidate their position of dominance in the industry. Such changes and their attendant economic pressures drive constraints in expenditure and inevitably direct innovation away from the search for new therapeutic plasma products and towards improvements in existing product processes. These improvements are generally targeted at increasing yield, and most notably have focused on enhancing the yield of intravenous immunoglobulin products. These products are now the driver of the industry and prices have doubled in recent years. Interestingly however, despite the significant increases in both yield and unit selling price, the registered clinical indications for these products remain essentially the same, notwithstanding a significant body of medical evidence for their effectiveness in a wide range of neurological and other disorders. This apparent reluctance to conduct clinical trials for new indications may reflect a belief that a

[2] The section on Plasma Products kindly provided by personal communication with Neil Goss (formerly with CSL Bioplasma).

recombinant intravenous immunoglobulin, or at least monoclonal antibody therapy for some specific indications, may be nearing reality. It is true that recombinant clotting factors have largely replaced their plasma derived equivalents in the developed world and the Japanese are now producing a recombinant albumin. A fully recombinant intravenous immunoglobulin is however quite a different challenge. Alternatively, the lack of clinical trials focused on new indications for intravenous immunoglobulin may reflect a variety of other factors including: the cost of these trials and their subsequent registration, the fact that the products are already used "off-label" for non-registered indications, the existing restricted supply of the products caused by the economics of the industry that cannot justify producing intravenous immunoglobulin alone from plasma, the fact that any company conducting clinical trails could suffer from the "pioneer syndrome" - incurring significant costs for the trials and registration while failing to gain an exclusive right to exploit that indication and even making it considerably easier and cheaper for competitor companies to register a me-too indication for their own product. Whatever the reason, the reality is that in a marketplace where demand outstrips supply there is no commercial justification for any additional expenditure other than for the purpose of increasing yield.

While the demand for intravenous immunoglobulin has been increasing in the developed world, the burgeoning economies of China and India in particular have in recent years supported significantly increased demand for albumin and to a lesser extent for factor VIII. The need in these countries has been for existing plasma products rather than new products and therefore there has been little pressure or incentive for new product research and development in the plasma fractionation industry. Thus even in a period of considerable commercial activity and economic prosperity there appears to be little incentive for the major fractionators to conduct research into new plasma products. Perhaps this will change in the future as modern plants come on stream in the developing world and the opportunity to explore the therapeutic potential of new plasma products presents itself.

QUALITY MANAGEMENT

Quality Management is an extremely important part of Transfusion Medicine. This is both at the production of blood products and at the time of transfusion.

It is not without some controversy or frequent analysis and discussion.

How much is too much? Is it possible to have too much [23,24]?

Is at least some of the Quality Management that is introduced (at least or in part) based on political motives rather than the outcome for the patient?

Should Quality Management be focused on the issues that are of major risk and extreme outcomes rather than have an "all encompassing" direction?

Is it possible that extreme demands that can be required by a very emphasis on Quality Management and documentation actually take the focus off some of the critical issues that are high risk and high probability?

There is also the very clear acknowledgement that the increase in regulations and limitation that are applied to donor requirements and product requirements have had some influence on the availability of blood products [25].

Finally, there is also the requirement to recall product that may be of very low risk. This can in some situations have the potential to lead to product shortages that almost certainly will have a higher risk than having the very low risk product still available.

Of course all of these issues are out of line with most of the official dogma relating to Quality Systems and the Quality management that is accepted and expected to be applied to all aspects of Transfusion

Throughout the history of transfusion, there have been many advances that have been made available or have been stimulated by some significant adversity – quite often during war [26-34].

It is possible that this book had its origin during a period immediately following the Bali bombing amongst the negotiations and the production of blood products and eventual outcome from the use of those blood products on the Australians who were unfortunate enough to be almost half of the victims.

In 2000 three bombs were detonated in Bali. This had devastating implications for 168 people in Bali. 80 of them were Australians. After immediate treatment in Bali and some brief time in Darwin many of them were transferred to Perth, Western Australia.

During the first briefing at Royal Perth Hospital it was suggested that those patients, who needed major burns surgery, should be provided with fresh, unrefrigerated whole blood. (This had previously been successfully used for several patients with major blood loss). It was going to be a challenge but the subsequent outcome was impressive.

It was at this time that the idea of this book was probably born. It wasn't realized at the time but in hindsight it was clear that the message was that there were lessons that were learnt during that period – not least of which that there is often an opportunity to have the conviction to try something a little unusual, always have the patients welfare at heart and to consult people with knowledge and experience – even if it doesn't necessarily follow the classical or current thinking.

This book is designed to not necessarily follow the convention. It will not answer all of the questions. Hopefully it is going to stimulate and question – and present some alternatives when considering production and transfusion.

It is an opportunity to hear the view of many individuals who are expert in their particular field of the business of transfusion - who have many years and extensive experience in Blood Transfusion.

How do we bring these requirements together? How do we find some middle ground or get agreement for the best possible option?

Although it is a part of Medicine that has been inundated with classical/historic expectations and culture. There is a plethora of guidelines, definitions of appropriateness, audits. It is not the aim to in anyway discard or devalue these essential requirements.

However, I hope the main message that will come from this book is:

TRANSFUSION – THINK ABOUT IT!

REFERENCES

[1] Reyes G, Nuche JM, Sarraj A, et al. Bloodless Cardiac Surgery in Jehovah's Witnesses: Outcome compared with a Control Group. *Revista Espanola de cardiologia* 2007;60(7): 727-731.

[2] Viele MK, Weiskopf RB. What can we learn about the need for transfusion from patients who refuse blood? The experience with Jehovah's Witnesses. *Transfusion* 1994;34:396-401.

[3] Council of Europe Guide to the Preparation, *Use and Quality Assurance of Blood Components* (14th Edition; 2008).

[4] *Therapeutic Goods A*ct (1989).

[5] *ANZSBT Guidelines for pretransfusion laboratory practice* (2007).

[6] *ANZSBT Administration Guidelines* (2004).

[7] *NHMRC/ASBT Clinical practice guidelines* (2001).

[8] NHMRC/ASBT . Clinical Practice Guidelines on the Use of Blood Components (red blood cells, platelets, fresh frozen plasma, cryoprecipitate). Endorsed September 2001. Published by Commonwealth of Australia 2002.

[9] The Stationery Office (TSO), London (UK) (Publisher). *Guidelines for the Blood Transfusion Services in the United Kingdom* (7th Edition 2005.

[10]Keung CY, Smith KR, Savoia HF, Davidson AJ. An audit of transfusion of red blood cell units in pediatric anesthesia. *Paediatr Anaesth.*2009 (19): 320 -328.

[11]Qureshi H, Lowe D, Dobson P, Grant-Casey J, Parris E, Dalton D, Hickling K, Waller F, Howell C, Murphy MF, National Blood Service/Royal College of Physicians National Comparative Audit of Blood Transfusion programme. National comparative audit of the use of platelet transfusions in the UK. *Transfus Clin Biol.* 2007 (14): 509-513.

[12]Jackson GN, Snowden CA, Indrikovos AJ. A prospective audit program to determine blood component transfusion appropriateness at a large university hospital: a 5 year experience. *Transfusion Medicine Reviews*. 2008 (22):154 – 161.

[13]Mirzamani N, Molana A, Poorani E. Evaluation of appropriate usage of frozen plasma: Results of a regional audit in Iran. *Transfusion Apheresis Science*. 2009 (40): 109 – 113.

[14]Wang JK, Klein HG. Red blood cell transfusion in the treatment and management of anaemia: the search for the elusive transfusion trigger. *Vox Sang* (Epub 2009 Aug 4).

[15]Perkins JG, Andrew CP, Spinella PC, Blackbourne LH, Grathwohl KW, Repine TB, Ketchum L, Waterman P, Lee RE, Beekley AC, Sebesta JA, Shorr AF, Wade CE, Holcomb JB. *J Trauma*. 2009 (66) (Suppl 4): S77 – S84.

[16]Adukauskiene D, Kinderyte A, Veikutiene A. Indications for platelet transfusion. Medicina (Kaunas) 2008 (40): 905 – 909.

[17]Sperry JL, Ochoa JB, Gunn SR, Alarcon LH, Minei JP, Cuschieri J, Rosengart MR, Maier RV, Billiar TR, Peitzman AB, Moore EE, Inflammation the Host Response to Injury Investigators. *J Trauma*. 2008 (65): 986 – 993.

[18]Wallis JP. Red cell transfusion triggers. *Transfusion Apheresis Science*. 2008 (39): 151 – 154.

[19]Alport EC, Callum JL, Nahimiak S, Eurich B, Hume HA. Cryoprecipitate use in 25 Canadian hospitals: commonly used outside of the published guidelines. *Transfusion*. 2008 (48): 2122 – 2127.

[20]Ohsaka A, Abe K, Ohsawa T, Miyake N, Sugita S, Tojima I. A computer-assisted transfusion management system and changed transfusion practices contribute to appropriate management of blood components. *Transfusion*. 2008 (48): 1730 – 1738.

[21]von Lindern JS, Brand A. The use of blood products in perinatal medicine. *Semin Fetal Neonatal Medicine*. 2008 (13): 272 – 281.

[22]Farrugia A. The regulatory pendulum in transfusion medicine. *Transfusion Medicine Reviews*. 2002 (16): 273 – 282.

[23]van Reeuwijk LP, Houba VJ. *Guidelines for quality management in soil and plant laboratories*, Daya Press, 2001.

[24]Kendrick Tom. Results Without Authority: Controlling a Project When the Team Doesn't Report to You. *American Management Association (AMACOM)* 2006. New York

[25]Cobain TJ. Fresh Blood Product Manufacture, Issue and Use: A chain of Diminishing Returns? *Transfusion Medicine Reviews* 2004, 18 (4):279-292.

[26]Stansbury LG, Hess JR. Blood Transfusion in World War I: The roles of Lawrence Bruce Robertson and Oswald Hope Robertson in the "Most Important Medical Advance of the War". *Transfusion Medicine Reviews*. 2009 (23): 232 – 236.

[27]Strauss RG. Elmer L. DeGowin, MD: Blood Transfusions in War and Peace. *Transfusion Medicine Reviews*. 2006 (20): 165 – 168.

[28]Spinella PC. Warm fresh whole blood transfusion for severe hemorrhage: US military and potential civilian applications. *Critical Care Medicine*. 2008 (36 (7 Suppl)): S340 – S345.

[29]Propper BW, Rasmussen TE, Davidson SB, Vandenberg SL, Clouse WD, Burkhardt GE, Gifford SM, Johannigman JA. Surgical response to multiple casualty incidents following single explosive events. *Annals of Surgery*. 2009 (250): 311 – 315.

[30]Spinella PC, Perkins JG, Grathwohl KW, Beekley AC, Holcomb JB. Warm fresh whole blood is independently associated with improved survival for patients with combat-related traumatic injuries. *J Trauma*. 2009 (66) (4 Suppl): S69 – S76.

[31]Nessen SC, Cronk DR, Edens J, Eastridge BJ, Little TR, Windsor J, Blackbourne LH, Holcomb JB. US Army two surgeon teams operating in remote Afghanistan-an evaluation of split-based Forward Surgical Team Operations. *J Trauma* 2009 (66) (4 Suppl): S37 – S47.

[32]Dunne JR, Hawksworth JS, Stojadinovic A, Gage F, Tadaki DK, Perdue PW, Forsberg J, Davis T, Denbile JW, Brown TS, Elster EA. Perioperative blood transfusion in combat casualties: a pilot study. *J Trauma* 2009 (66) (4 Suppl): S150 – S156.

[33]Miller RD. Massive blood transfusion: the impact of Vietnam military data on modern civilian transfusion medicine. *Anesthesiology* 2009 (110): 1412 – 1416.

[34]Zarychanski R, Ariano RE, Paunovic B, Bell DD. Historical perspectives in critical care medicine: blood transfusion, intravenous fluids, inotropes/vasopressors, and antibiotics. *Critical Care Clinics* 2009 (25): 201 – 220.

In: Transfusion - Think About It
Editor: Trevor J. Cobain
ISBN 978-1-61668-969-8

Chapter 1

DECISION MAKING IN TRANSFUSION MEDICINE

James P. Isbister*
University of Sydney, New South Wales, Australia.

ABSTRACT

Blood transfusion has had a central role in modern medicine. In more recent times the question is more frequently asked if transfusion of allogeneic blood/products are justified or required. This may have, in part, been driven by HIV and other infectious agents being associated with transfusion but is also related to improved data relating to alternatives to transfusion and more scrutiny of transfusion relating to cost and efficiency.

It is reasonable to expect that the question will be ask if allogeneic transfusion can be minimized or avoided by appropriate diagnosis and management with alternatives and not regarding transfusion as the default decision..

The principles for the practice of allogeneic transfusion can be based in general terms on evidence relating to the scientific basis for the therapeutic decision to transfuse or not. It is also based on the ethical responsibility to the patient receiving the transfusion, the donor of the blood and the general community. In addition the economic responsibilities relating to the cost effectiveness and value in following a particular direction relating to the use of blood products must be considered.

These directions will also mean that alternatives will be considered and may be used before transfusion and that the patient or responsible relative will be included and informed during this decision making process.

* Correspondence concerning this article should be addressed to: James P. Isbister, Department of Haematology and Transfusion Medicine, Royal North Shore Hospital of Sydney, Faculty of Medicine, University of Sydney, St Leonards, New South Wales. Australia 2065; e mail: JIsbiste@med.usyd.edu.au.

Introduction

Blood transfusion has had a central role in the development and practice of modern medicine. It is only in recent years that blood transfusion is no longer regarded as essential in a wide range of clinical settings, indeed, it is now possible for the majority of uncomplicated elective surgery to be conducted without allogeneic blood component therapy. Experience with Jehovah Witness patients who refuse transfusion on religious grounds has questioned the assumption that allogeneic transfusion is a prerequisite for the success of many major surgical procedures [2]. Several reported series of elective surgery in Jehovah Witness patients indicate less morbidity, shorter intensive care unit and hospital lengths of stay than for matched patients receiving red cell transfusions. Perhaps of even more importance is the evidence that these patients are better prepared for surgery, have less bleeding and better postoperative haemoglobin levels and recovery times [3]. The corollary of this is that these patients receive a different (ie better) standard of clinical care pointing to a more patient and disease focused (ie problem-based) clinical practice.

The recognition in the 1980's that AIDS was a viral disease that could be transmitted by allogeneic blood transfusion resulted in a resurgence of interest in methods for minimising exposure to allogeneic blood products. Blood transfusion has commonly not been regarded in the same light as other risk/benefit decisions in clinical medicine. Assiduous attention to accurate diagnosis, due consideration of therapeutic options and their potential hazards are as essential to blood component therapy as it is with any other medical interventions. Blood transfusion is a process within overall clinical management with short-term surrogate endpoints that in many circumstances have not be shown to correlate with improvement in clinical outcomes. In many clinical conditions in which blood component therapy plays a key role the evidence for benefit is substantial and relatively easy to balance against the risk of potential hazards. The management of critical haemorrhage, haemophilia, prevention of RhD haemolytic disease of the newborn, immunoglobulin therapy for antibody deficiency states are all examples.

Although appropriate endpoints may be achieved in terms of measurable parameters or immediate clinical response evidence is required that traditionally used surrogate endpoints are relevant in relation to the final outcome for the patient. There are numerous appropriate clinical or laboratory endpoints within clinical management pivotal to a successful final outcome, but there are others where dogma rather than evidence has dominated clinical practice. The HIV crisis brought into focus that there were many transfusion practices exposing patients to potential hazards without convincing evidence for identifiable short or long-term benefit/s. Many patients contracted HIV from allogeneic transfusions that, on retrospective review, were inappropriate.

When considering decision making in transfusion medicine are we asking the right question? In giving primacy to clinical practice guidelines for blood component therapy we are probably falling into the common trap of starting with an answer before the question has been clearly considered. A similar error is commonly made in marketing when a business does not clearly identify in which business it is operating. This point became part of marketing folklore following a landmark article in the Harvard Business Review "Marketing Myopia" in 1960 [4]. In this article Levitt makes the point that, in the early history of railroads the tycoons considered they were in the business of making railroads, when in fact they were in the transport business. As a result they were not able to adapt appropriately when other means of transport became available. By analogy transfusion medicine is in the business of helping to improve clinical outcomes, not primarily to provide "blood, the gift of life". Clinical outcomes are improved by evidence-based diagnosis and therapy of diseases in which blood component therapy may have a role to play, if alternative therapies are not available.

From the haematological perspective the primary responsibility of clinicians is to manage a patient's own blood as a precious and unique human resource that should not be wasted and to consider donor sourced allogeneic blood components when there is no alternative. This more recent concept of patient blood management is increasingly focusing on the patient and their clinical problems as well as giving them a greater role and responsibility in their own clinical management [5]. This evolution towards a patient blood management philosophy in clinical practice, is in contrast to behavior-based transfusion management as the main focus. Parallel to this paradigm shift back to the patient is greater emphasis on clinical decision making based on sound scientific evidence. Benchmarking studies in orthopaedic surgery have been revealing in highlighting major differences in red cell transfusion practices for comparable patient groups [6]. There are also difficulties in explaining significant variations in the red cell transfusion rates per head of population within individual countries and internationally.

PRINCIPLES OF PRACTICE IN TRANSFUSION MEDICINE

In general decision making in blood component therapy is no different from other therapeutic decisions, why, "in general"? Patients think blood transfusion is special and beneficial, but have difficulty accepting small risks they can't control. Clinicians think blood is ordinary, take blood transfusion for granted, benefit is assumed and risks regarded as minimal. Funders and Governments view blood as a commodity and transfusion medicine as an expensive support service which should be regulated and funded in a "McDonaldised" manner. Blood donors believe their non remunerated voluntary contribution of blood is a gift to the community that will be used appropriately and safely. Clinicians and funders have an ethical responsibility that the donors gift, given in trust, will be managed and used appropriately for the benefit of the greatest number of patients in need. Blood from voluntary, non remunerated, blood donors, cannot be regarded as a pharmaceutical, ie is a commodity in contrast to blood components from paid donors or of recombinant origin. The three E's triangle of clinical practice should be uppermost in the clinician's mind and the best efforts made to keep the triangle equilateral.

- **Evidence**: The scientific basis for therapeutic decisions
- **Ethics**: Ethical responsibilities towards patients, donors and the community (equity)
- **Economics**: Cost effectiveness and value for money in the broadest sense

Unfortunately, these three E's commonly become surrounded by emotions and the triangle becomes unbalanced.

In most circumstances allogeneic blood transfusion is required for haematological deficiencies until the basic disease process can be corrected. Therapy may control the effects of a deficiency or used prophylactically to prevent or minimise problems. In general, allogeneic blood transfusion should not be regarded as the first line of therapy for patients with haemopoietic deficiency or potential deficits. In many clinical contexts, especially where there is clinical uncertainty transfusion has been a default decision with benefit assumed and risks commonly inadequately assessed. Accumulating evidence from observation data and randomised controlled trials is incriminating transfusion of labile blood components (red cell and platelet concentrates and fresh frozen plasma) as independent risk factors for adverse clinical outcomes. This evidence demands a more precautionary approach to transfusion and better evidence for benefit and improved clinical outcomes. A broad search of the Medline database for the terms [transfusion AND risk] and [transfusion AND benefit] returned a ratio of 5 to 1 publications. Recent clinical audit studies have highlighted that most red cell transfusions administered to stable anaemic patients contravene current clinical practice guidelines and are unlikely to be of benefit to the patient. In a recent editorial, Charlton, editor-in-chief of Medical Hypothesis, has coined the term "zombie science" for the perpetuation of beliefs and clinical practices that cannot be substantiated by real science [7]. This is perhaps the case with the use of the labile blood components. Even more provocative is the author's assertion, *"On the other hand, when a branch of science based on phoney theories is serving a useful but non-scientific purpose it may be kept-going by continuous transfusions of cash from those whose interests it serves"*.

For the majority of patients it should be possible to minimise requirements for allogeneic blood components or to correct, manage or tolerate the effects of deficiencies in the haematopoietic system without transfusion. This is particularly the case if the deficiency is reversible in the longer term. It is important to acknowledge that the majority of blood component transfusions are temporising and have no long-term benefit *per se*. Additionally, most indicators for benefit are surrogate makers of efficacy and evidence that these surrogates correlate with a better clinical outcome for the patient in many circumstances is weak and commonly based on accepted dogma. If benefit cannot be predicted and allogeneic blood avoided the potential hazards need not be considered, a point made on many occasions by plaintiff lawyers in transfusion transmitted HIV and Hepatitis medical negligence cases. There is no defence when a patient suffers major morbidity or mortality from an inappropriate or non-indicated therapy. It is not unreasonable for a cross examining barrister to ask; *"Doctor, what clinical benefit were you anticipating to achieve from the transfusion that gave my client HIV?"* Transfusion decision making can be difficult and debate continues regarding the indications for transfusion, especially in relationship to the labile allogeneic blood components. However, if you start with the problem you may find a way out, but if you start with the solution you risk being locked out.

The Pre-emptive Questions

In addressing the role of allogeneic blood transfusion in the management of individual patients there are several questions requiring consideration:

- What is the timeframe of the clinical decision making process?
- Is it an elective decision?
- What is the haematological defect?
- What is the most appropriate therapy for the patient?

- Have specific patient related additional risk factors been identified?
- Are there alternatives to allogeneic blood component transfusion available?
- What blood component is indicated and from where should it be obtained?
- What are the potential hazards of the blood component therapy?
- Can the risk of potential adverse effects be avoided or minimised?
- How should the blood component be administered and monitored?
- What is the global cost of the haemotherapy?
- Is the patient fully informed of the medical decisions?

What are the Requirements for a Safe and Effective Transfusion?

- There must be a clearly defined indication and anticipated benefit
- There must be accurate patient identification for compatibility testing and administration
- Provision of adequate amounts and quality of the component/s
- Communication of benefits and risk to the patient/relatives
- Identification and appropriate management of high-risk patients
- The transfusion should not be associated with any ill effects
- Appropriate handling, administration and monitoring of the blood component
- Awareness of possible transfusion-related complications
- Early recognition and prompt action in relation to transfusion associated adverse events
- Appropriate documentation of the indication and administration in the clinical records
- If the decision to transfusion is outside the clinical practice guidelines the reason must be included in the clinical records.
- There should be input into quality assurance programmes

Evidence-based Transfusion Medicine

With scientific evidence as one of the points of the 3Es triangle, evidenced-based medicine (EBM) is increasingly influencing the practice of transfusion medicine. On the surface this appears appropriate and laudable, however there are problems when EBM is narrowly defined and practiced with almost religious fervour. EBM should not be restricted to the uncritical clinical application of frequentist statistical analysis from randomised clinical trials, no matter how good the trials may be.

The traditional approach to clinical decision-making is to identify the patient's problem (ie diagnosis) and consider appropriate therapy. When in doubt one consults references (textbook or journals) and/or asks a respected colleague/s for advice. A decision is ultimately made for which the clinician accepts responsibility. This classical approach is observer dependent in contrast to the epidemiologically numerically and analytically focused evidenced based medicine approach advocating a more proscriptive and objective process to arrive at a decision. With the EBM approach an appropriate clinical question is formulated, a literature search conducted with the selection and critically appraisal of relevant articles and the conclusions applied to a specific patient. This is a more objective and scientific approach and places more emphasis on "the evidence", assuming there is good evidence. A good clinician today practices a balance between the classical and EBM approaches which continues to place emphasis on clinical judgement +/- the "art of medicine".

As with all modern medical therapy, blood component therapy presupposes an understanding of disease in terms of pathophysiology, definition, classification, diagnosis, indicators of severity and prediction of the natural history of untreated and treated disease. With many clinical disorders where blood component therapy may have a role the disease or problem is well understood in the above terms (eg haemophilia, rhesus haemolytic disease). However, with other disorders our understanding can only be regarded as rudimentary (eg the role of red cell concentrates in the management of stable patients with anaemia). Clinical decision making and therapy have analytical, numerical, clinical and application aspects that require consideration, individually and collectively. To achieve these ends the questions in figure 1 should be addressed during the course of a patient clinical management.

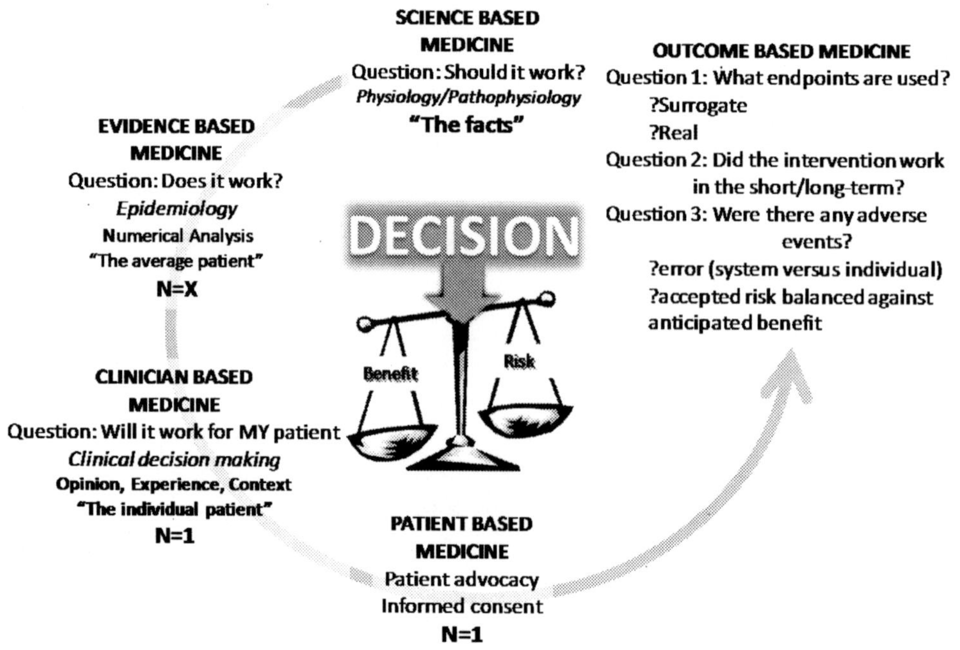

Figure 1. The process of modern scientific medical practice addressing the question of the efficacy and safety of a clinical intervention. This model does not specifically take into account economic and ethical principles that are also central issues in modern medicine.

This approach may seem contrary to the now commonly accepted "levels of evidence" that are in the context of the numeral epidemiological approach and only applies to question 2 in the algorithm in figure 1.

1. Should the therapy be effective?

- Is the therapy logical on the basis of the current level of understanding of physiology and pathophysiology?

2. Is there evidence the therapy is effective and do the benefits outweigh the potential hazards?
    - What numeral experimental data is available to support efficacy and identify potential hazards? This is the "levels of evidence". Red cell transfusions have been "grandfathered" into clinical medicine not having to fulfill the regulatory requirements that are today demanded for new therapies to be introduced into medical practice (figure 2).

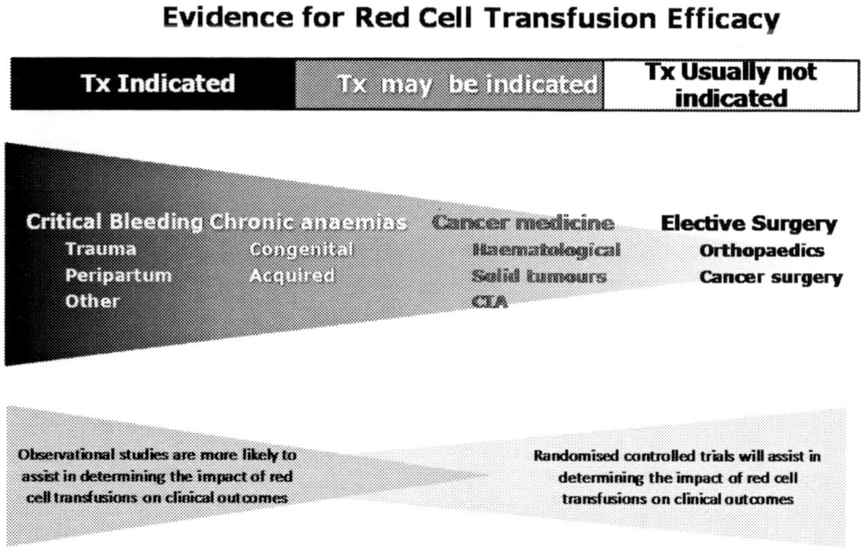

Figure 2. The efficacy and safety of red cell transfusions are now coming into question with clinical practice guidelines more opinion-based than evidence-based. This figure illustrates how the issues of red cell transfusion efficacy and safety may be addressed. CIA = Chemotherapy Induced Anaemia.

3. Will the therapy be effective for the individual patient in question?
    - This is the context depended issue in clinical decision making. Does the patient have any specific considerations (eg risk factors) that may impact on efficacy or risk? Would the patient be eligible for entry into the clinical trial on which the evidence for the decision is being made? Are there broader psychosocial considerations to be incorporated into the clinical decision making process.
4. Following the therapeutic intervention, has the anticipated outcome been achieved?
    - What parameters are being used to assess efficacy and complications in the short and long-term? If these parameters are surrogates for the anticipated outcome what evidence is there for their correlation with the outcome?
5. In the event that there is an adverse outcome, has it been appropriately identified and managed?

- Was the adverse outcome an accepted possibility and was it diagnosed and managed appropriately? Were pre-emptive measures taken to avoid or minimise the risk of the adverse outcome?
- Was the adverse outcome the result of an error in management and has a root cause analysis been carried out?

Figure 3 illustrates the "real World" of evidence based medicine.

At the risk of being over philosophical, the master clinician has a "handle" on what is known, what is thought to be known and what is not known. The master clinician also has a good understanding of the difference between data, information, knowledge and wisdom. When there is sound understanding of the physiology and pathophysiology, question two and the levels of evidence will be bypassed. For example, when it was recognised that AIDS was a virally related disease due to HIV transmitted by bodily fluids, including blood, a randomised controlled of infected allogeneic blood versus non-infected would never be done, let alone accepted by any ethics committee. Similarly, when the ABO blood groups were discovered a randomised controlled clinical trial of *in vitro* crossmatched blood and uncrossmatched blood would never be performed.

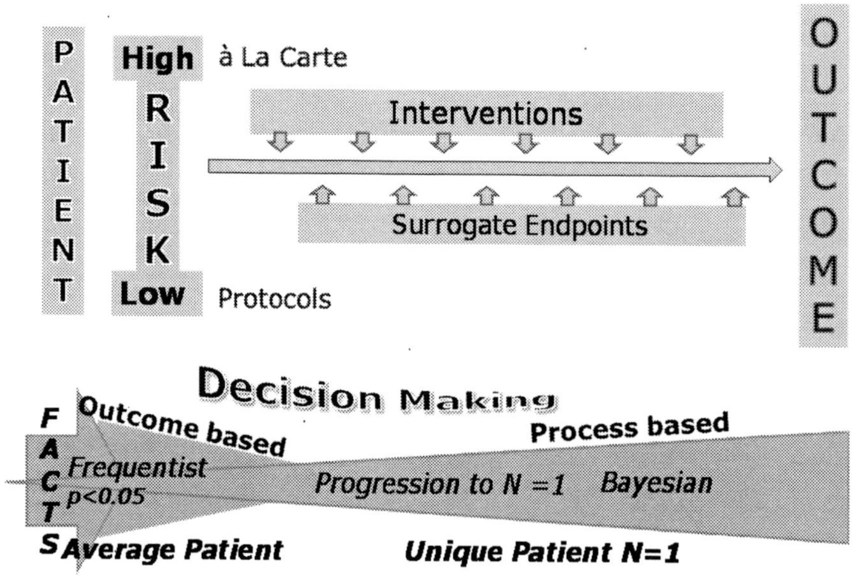

Figure 3. The "real World" of evidence based clinical practice. A unique patient (ie N = 1) presents to a clinician who makes an initial diagnosis and management decisions on the basis known facts (pathophysiology) and knowledge from numerical analysis (ie frequentist statistics, N = x, and levels of evidence). The clinician uses this information to progress from decision making on the basis of an average patient to the context and specific characteristics of the patient under consideration (process based analysis N = 1).

CLINICAL PRACTICE GUIDELINES

Clinical guidelines are systematically developed statements to assist decision making about appropriate healthcare for specific clinical circumstances. In the past there has been a tendency to develop guidelines around specific therapeutic interventions in contrast to focusing on the clinical problem, ie the answer has taken priority over the question. This has been the case with several aspects of blood component therapy, particularly the indications for the labile (fresh) blood components. As mentioned it is ironic that more is known about the hazards of the labile blood components than their evidence for benefit in improving clinical outcomes.

Clinical Guidelines are of Greatest Value when:-

- it is possible to make a clear diagnosis and predict the outcome
- physiology and pathophysiology is well understood
- there is good quality evidence for effective therapy
- the potential hazards of therapy are known and likelihood for occurrence quantified (ie risk)
- there is variability between clinicians, hospitals and countries in management for a clearly defined clinical entity.
- there is predictable use of resources and a potential for consistent measurable outcomes in terms of efficacy, complications and costs
- There may be difficulties with clinical guidelines when:-
    - the evidence is incorrect or poorly researched
    - they have been developed by narrow interest group/s
    - the pathophysiology is poorly understood or falls outside the guidelines
    - there are medico legal implications
    - there are unique patient variables (risk factors) impacting on clinical decision making
    - there are hidden agendas of policy makers, ie the prime consideration is reducing costs

PATIENT INFORMED CONSENT

Ensuring patient-focused informed consent is a well established and legal requirement in clinical practice, blood transfusion should be no exception.

Patients and their relatives assume they will receive competently practiced evidence based medicine that will be customized to their needs. They naturally assume that they are unique and personalized medicine is increasingly society's expectation. (figure 4).

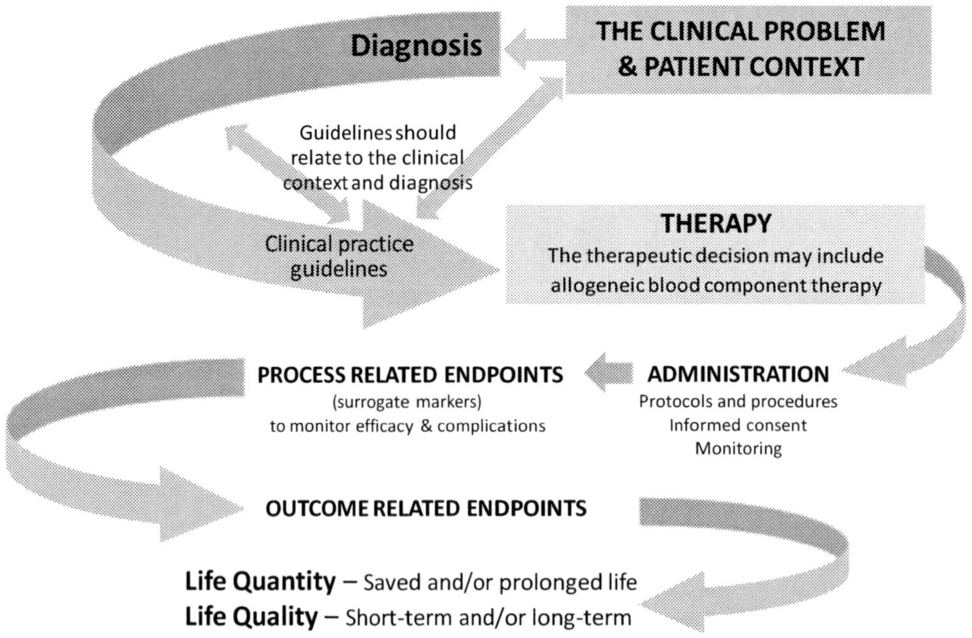

Figure 4. The basic principles clinical practice guidelines, focusing on the patient with a clinical problem rather than centering around the therapeutic intervention.

Randy Pausch eloquently summarises these perception and expectations in his recent book "The Last Lecture" when writing about his newborn son being admitted to neonatal intensive care. "*Dylan was sent to the neonatal intensive care unit. I came to recognize that parents with babies there needed very specific reassurances from doctors and nurses. They did a wonderful job of simultaneously communicating two dissonant things. In so many words, they told parents that, 1) your child is special and we understand that his medical needs are unique and 2) don't worry, we've had a million babies like yours come through here.*"

Considering allogeneic blood transfusion can be regarded as a transplant procedure. It is essential that a patient understands clearly what benefits are to be anticipated from the transfusion and the potential hazards to which they are being exposed. The medical decision making processes have already been outlined and there needs to be documentation of the reasons for transfusion in the clinical records and the fact there has been a discussion with the patient or their representative.

From the patient perspective it is reasonable that they are encouraged to have a checklist [8]:

1. Do you understand why you need a blood transfusion?
2. Have the risks of transfusion been explained?
3. Have alternatives been discussed?
4. Have all your questions been answered?

The Society for the Advancement of Blood Management (SABM) have a list of questions patients are advised to asked their doctor [9]:

1. Will I need a transfusion? If so, why?
2. What are the risks involved with blood transfusions?

3. What are the risks if I choose to minimize or avoid blood transfusions?
4. Will I need iron, vitamins or medications to increase my blood count for this surgery?
5. If I do need a transfusion, how will it affect my recovery time?

Recognising and Managing Adverse Transfusion Outcomes

Figure 5 is an algorithm approach to awareness, diagnosis and management of adverse reactions to allogeneic blood transfusion.

When there is an adverse outcome identified as being related to blood transfusion it is important to do a root cause analysis to understand the underlying reasons and possibilities for future risk management and prevention (figure 6).

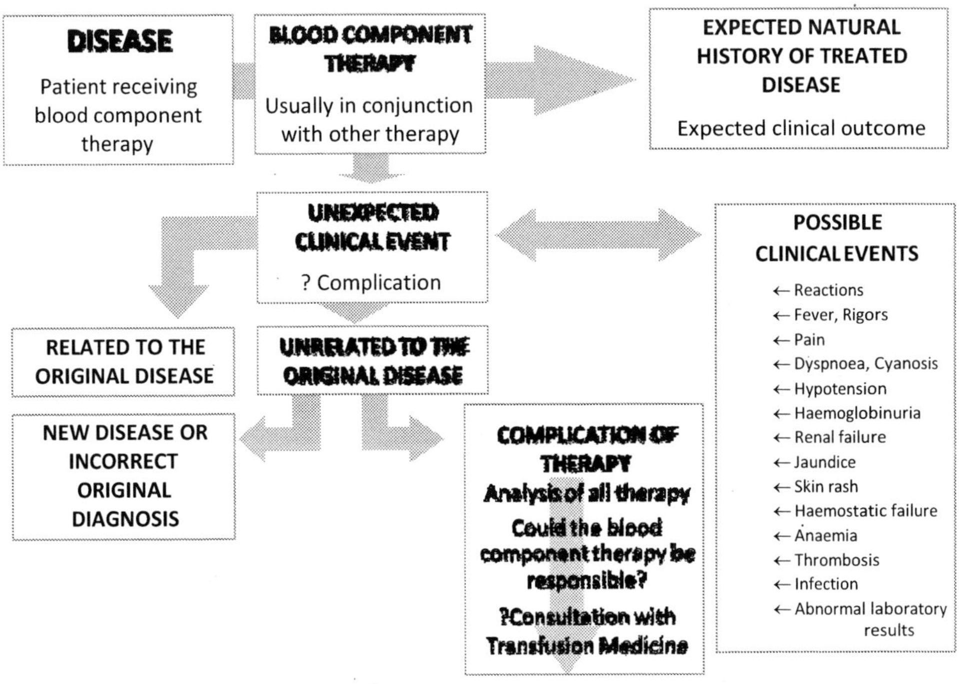

Figure 5. Algorithm for assessing and diagnosing adverse events that may be related to allogeneic blood transfusion.

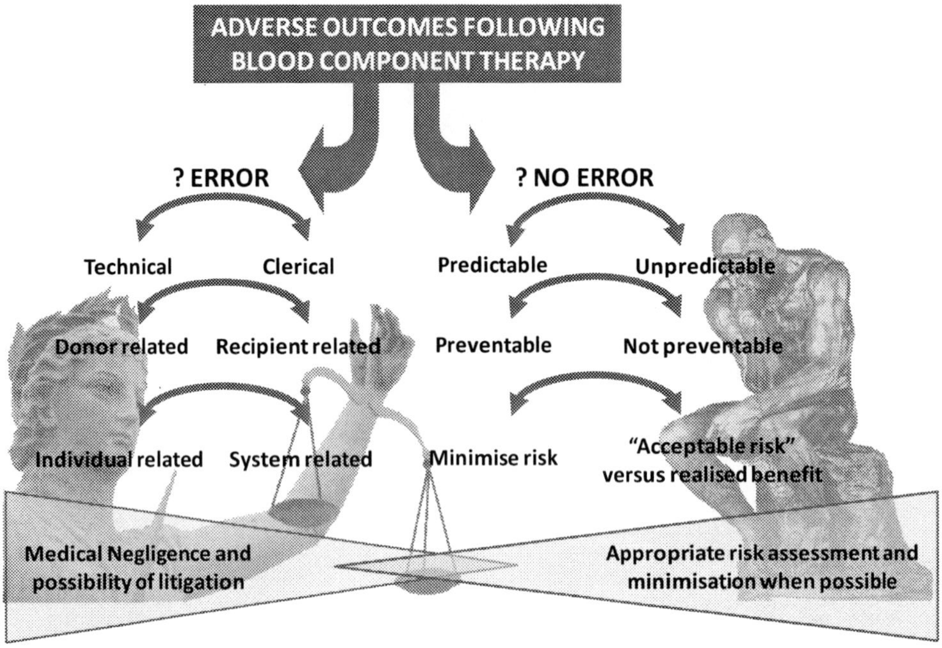

Figure 6. An algorithm approach for responding to an identified and analysed adverse outcome following blood transfusion.

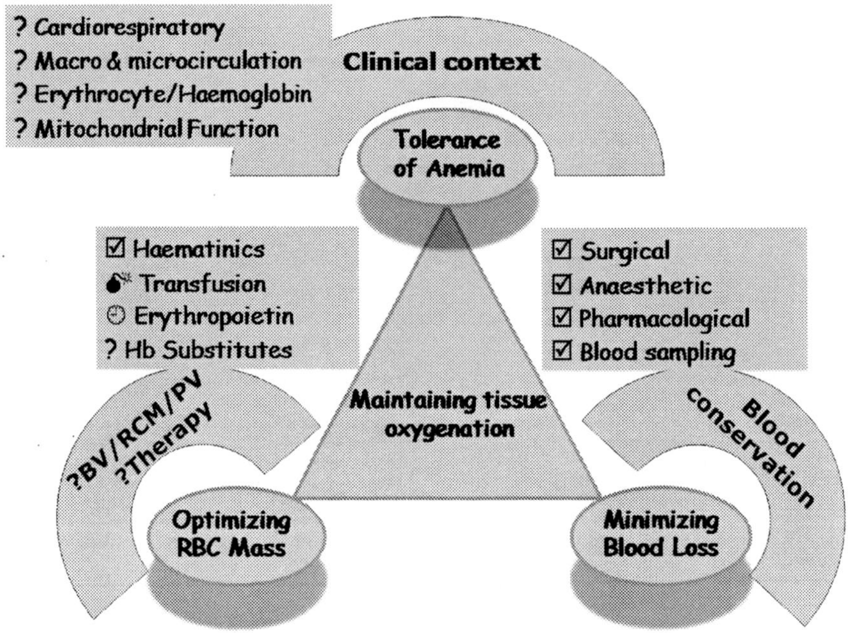

Figure 7. The three "pillars" for minimising/avoiding red cell transfusions.

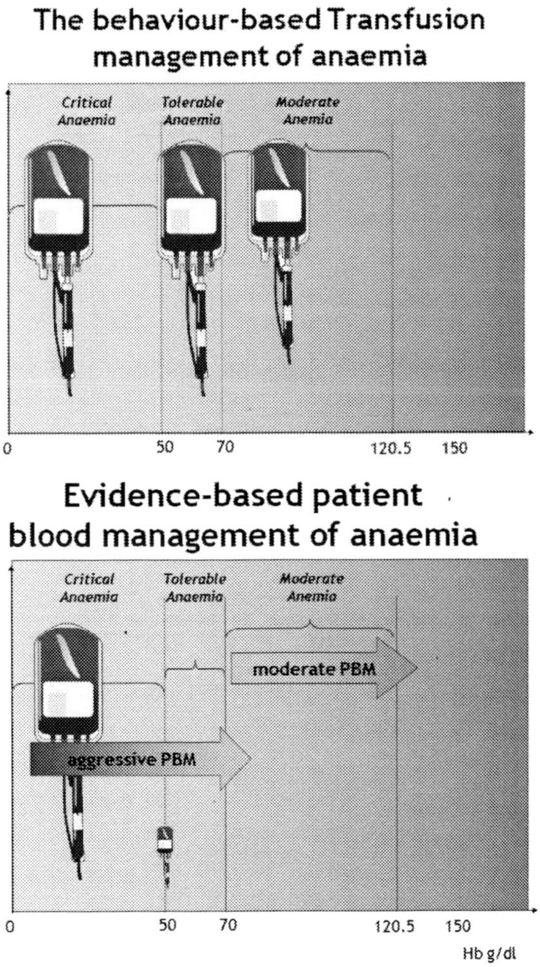

Figure 8. Red cell transfusion has been the traditional approach to the management of anaemia in the short-term. Anaemia is a defect in oxygen availability and delivery in which red cell transfusion may be appropriate therapy, but should not be the default decision. Red cell transfusion for correction of critical anaemia in a stable patient is acceptable standard of care. In the range of tolerable and moderate anaemia, red cell transfusion should not be regarded as the default therapy.

General Principles in Deciding when to use Labile Blood Components

A comprehensive review of guidelines for the use of all blood components is beyond the scope of this chapter and the reader is directed to numerous review and resources available. By focusing on the clinical problem the use of blood components should generally be a last resort option. Figures 7,8 & 9 illustrate with the example of anaemia an algorithmic approach to diagnosis and clinical management.

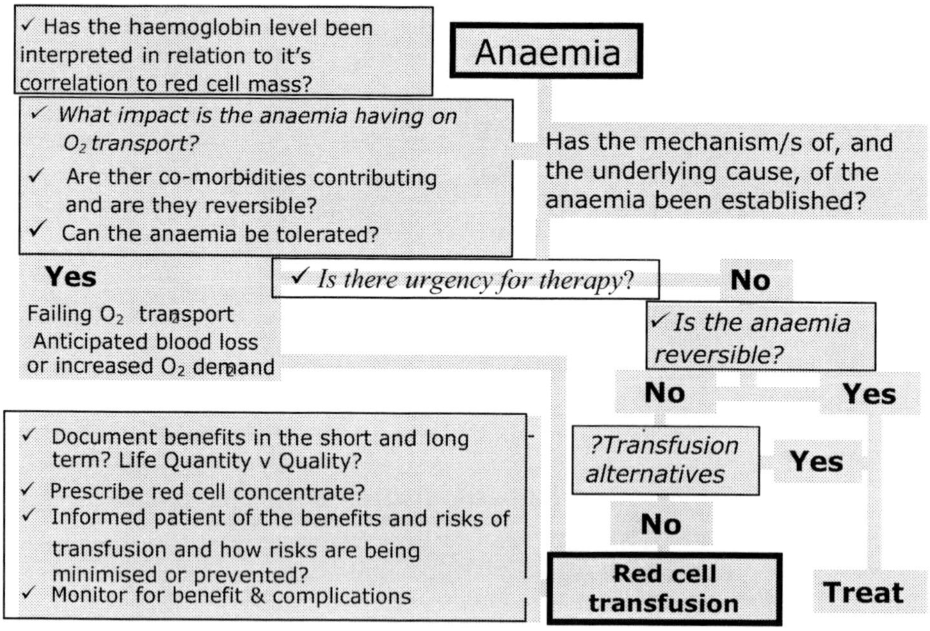

Figure 9. An algorithm for the management of anaemia with red cell transfusion as the last option, not the initial default decision.

Postscript: A Poignant Message from the History of Blood Transfusion

> *"Clinicians would be less confident in the safety of blood, and therefore more eclectic in its use, if they kept in mind the many possible weak links in the chain. In the hands of experts it is virtually safe, and very valuable; but there is little doubt that today, many deaths supposed to have occurred "in spite of transfusion" have really been caused by it. In fact, there are few risks in transfusion when the doctor fails to insert a needle or cannula into a vein; they begin to mount once he succeeds."*

I.H. Milner *The Lancet* [1].

Further Reading

Red cell concentrates [10,11,12,13,14].
Platelet concentrates [15,16].
Fresh frozen plasma and cryoprecipitate [17,18].
Intravenous immunoglobulin [19,20].
Critical bleeding [21].
Perioperative blood management [22]
Neonatal and paediatric transfusion medicine [23,24].

REFERENCES

[1] Milner IH. Foolproof Blood Transfusion. *The Lancet* 1949(July 30):217.

[2] Stamou SC, White T, Barnett S, Boyce SW, Corso PJ, Lefrak EA. Comparisons of cardiac surgery outcomes in Jehovah's versus Non-Jehovah's Witnesses. *The American journal of cardiology* 2006;98(9):1223-5.

[3] Reyes G, Nuche JM, Sarraj A, et al. Bloodless Cardiac Surgery in Jehovah's Witnesses: Outcomes Compared With a Control Group. *Revista espanola de cardiologia* 2007;60(7):727-31.

[4] Levitt T. Marketing Myopia. *Harvard Business Review* 1960(July-August):45-56.

[5] Spahn DR, Holger M, Hofmann A, Isbister J. Patient Blood Management: The Pragmatic Solution for the Problems with Blood Transfusions. *Anaesthesiology* 2008;109(6):951-3.

[6] Gombotz H, Rehak P, Shander A, Hofmann A. Blood use in elective surgery: the Austrian benchmark study. *Transfusion* 2007;47(8):1468-80.

[7] Charlton BG. Zombie science: a sinister consequence of evaluating scientific theories purely on the basis of enlightened self-interest. *Medical hypotheses* 2008;71(3):327-9.

[8] Clinical Excellence Commission. Patient Information Brochure: Blood Transfusion. http://wwwcechealthnswgovau/pdf/bloodwatch/blood_transfusionpdf NSW Health, Sydney Australia; Accessed March 2009.

[9] SABM. Patient's guide to blood management options. http://wwwsabmorg/professionals patientbrochure08pdf *Society for the Advancement of Blood Management*; Accessed March 2009.

[10] Spiess BD. Red Cell Transfusions and Guidelines: A Work in Progress. *Hematol Oncol Clin North Am* 2007;21(1):185-200.

[11] O'Riordan JM, Fitzgerald J, Smith OP, Bonnar J, Gorman WA. Transfusion of blood components to infants under four months: review and guidelines. *Irish medical journal* 2007;100(6):suppl 1-24 following 496.

[12] Debellis RJ. Anemia in critical care patients: Incidence, aetiology, impact, management, and use of treatment guidelines and protocols. *Am J Health Syst Pharm* 2007;64(3 Suppl 2):S14-21.

[13] Josephson CD, Su LL, Hillyer KL, Hillyer CD. Transfusion in the Patient With Sickle Cell Disease: A Critical Review of the Literature and Transfusion Guidelines. *Transfusion medicine reviews* 2007;21(2):118-33.

[14] Murphy MF, Wallington TB, Kelsey P, et al. Guidelines for the clinical use of red cell transfusions. *British Journal of Haematology* 2001;113(1):24-31.

[15] Bosly A, Muylle L, Noens L, et al. Guidelines for the transfusion of platelets. *Acta clinica Belgica* 2007;62(1):36-47.

[16] Guidelines for the use of platelet transfusions. *Br J Haematol* 2003;122(1):10-23.

[17] O'Shaughnessy DF, Atterbury C, Bolton Maggs P, et al. Guidelines for the use of fresh-frozen plasma, cryoprecipitate and cryosupernatant. *Br J Haematol* 2004;126(1):11-28.

[18] Hellstern P, Muntean W, Schramm W, Seifried E, Solheim BG. Practical guidelines for the clinical use of plasma. *Thrombosis research* 2002;107 Suppl 1:S53-7.

[19] Robinson P, Anderson D, Brouwers M, Feasby TE, Hume H. Evidence-based guidelines on the use of intravenous immune globulin for hematologic and neurologic conditions. *Transfusion medicine reviews* 2007;21(2 Suppl 1):S3-8.

[20]Anderson D, Ali K, Blanchette V, et al. Guidelines on the use of intravenous immune globulin for hematologic conditions. *Transfusion medicine reviews* 2007;21(2 Suppl 1):S9-56.

[21]British Committee for Standards in Haematology: Working Group: D.Stainsby SM, D.Thomas, J.Isaac and P.J.Hamilton. Guidelines on the management of massive blood loss. *British Journal of Haematology* 2006;135:634-41.

[22]Practice guidelines for perioperative blood transfusion and adjuvant therapies: an updated report by the American Society of Anaesthesiologists Task Force on Perioperative Blood Transfusion and Adjuvant Therapies. *Anaesthesiology* 2006;105(1):198-208.

[23]Gibson BE, Todd A, Roberts I, et al. Transfusion guidelines for neonates and older children. *Br J Haematol* 2004;124(4):433-53.

[24]Roseff SD, Luban NL, Manno CS. Guidelines for assessing appropriateness of paediatric transfusion. *Transfusion* 2002;42(11):1398-413.

In: Transfusion - Think About It
Editor: Trevor J. Cobain

ISBN 978-1-61668-969-8

Chapter 2

NATIONAL PRODUCTION PLANNING

Brenton Wylie
Gosford Hospital, Sydney, New South Wales, Australia.

ABSTRACT

Remarkably little has been published about planning a national blood supply. Its importance has only increased with the demands of modern medicine and the predicted decline in donors. For most situations the supply is really about fresh products given the open market or other particular systems for plasma products in most countries. For some however, including Australia, self sufficiency policy extends to fractionated products adding increased complexity to the planning process. Good planning in all cases flows from clearly stated national policies, known funding and resource bases, good systems for assessing current product demand, both met and unmet, and finally but not least good quality forecasts of factors impacting demand including population demographics, current and future clinical trends, product trends and developments in health infrastructure including new facilities and policies, for example drives to lower patient waiting lists.

INTRODUCTION

"If you don't know where you are going, any road will get you there"
- Lewis Carroll

There is remarkably little written in the literature about production supply planning at a national level [1,2]. At first glance it would seem to be a relatively straightforward exercise but a moment's consideration reveals the real complexities involved. Consider these questions. Who has ultimate responsibility for the adequacy of the supply? Is there an adequate supply now? Is there unmet demand and if so for which products and what is the gap? Is there any wastage of product currently and can this be addressed? How are population demographics likely to change in the future? How are the clinical practice changes and consequent product requirement likely to change? What new products and changes to existing products are likely, for example "artificial blood"? These are all important questions that will affect any planning process and for most of us the answers are either generally only partly known or at best the source of speculation! Generally the collection of good quality data especially on utilisation has also been a weakness for those trying to plan for the future [3].

Thus the task of planning a national blood supply is challenging to say the least. There are however some principles and basic steps that can be taken that should will enable planners to determine a reasonable path forward through the minefield. This chapter discusses ways forward through a review of the literature and this author's personal experience.

DRIVERS OF PRODUCTION-DEMAND

Probably the most fundamental parameter to ascertain is what product or products are driving the blood supply. This will vary from place to place but for most producers red cells will be the principal driver for fresh products. The role of platelets as a co-driver for production will vary dependant on overall demand but also the type of platelet product required. Historically platelet rich plasma platelets (PRP platelets) have been easily available as an ancillary product from whole blood collections, but the move towards buffycoat pools and especially single donor aphaeresis platelets has brought additional considerations and complexity to the planning process. This is particularly so at certain times of the year where a 5 day expiry can become problematic over public holiday periods. For some countries, including Australia, plasma products, principally intravenous immunoglobulin, act as an additional driver on supply. In this case in my experience a blood service can be faced with the immediate day to day problem of having red cells of each blood group but also the long term strategic problem is to ensure sufficient plasma is available for fractionation.

DEMAND PLANNING

As time management specialist Alan Lakein has said "planning is bringing the future into the present so that you can do something about it now". Fundamental to the exercise is getting the best idea you possibly can of product demand for the timeframe for which you are planning. Whilst demand planning needs to be applied to all products it is particularly relevant for the drivers of production.

Red Cell Demand

Red cell production is generally the central product for demand planning for fresh products. Planners should have a good idea of whether demand is being seen to be currently met by clinicians and others. If there is a perception of a current shortage in supply this needs to be defined and if possible quantified. In particular the difference between what may be viewed by some as the requirement needs to be tested against realistic needs for the system given the country's current level of health care delivery. A sobering lesson from my early career came when I found that the clinical group creating the greatest demand for better and fresher red cell product actually had an expiry rate considerably higher than any other similar sized institution! The problem wasn't so much the supply they were getting but their own management of this precious resource. Sazama has written an excellent review on the ethics of blood management [4].

How much is Enough?

Virtually all countries would like to have greater access to red cells so the question arises as to what level of supply should be enough especially as this product is likely to be driving their entire production system. A WHO reference has previously outlined the demand for blood donations based on a WHO study [5,6]. This can in turn be used as an indicator for the red cell supply needs in broad terms based on the stage of development of a particular country. The number of blood donations for a developed country was found to average 52 per 1000 but only 5 in middle-income countries and 1.5 in low-income countries. The ratio of donations to hospital admissions was also assessed and found to be 0.44, 0.33 and 0.25 for high, middle and low income countries respectively. In the same WHO reference Szilassy also looked at models assessing the number of donations a country may require, one using a figure based on 5% of the countries population and the other based of the total number of hospital beds in the country [7]. In reality in a developed country red cell utilisation rates may vary considerably. Cobain recently reported rates between 28 and 54 per 1000 [8].

In assessing demand a number of questions need to be addressed.

What is the historical trend? Red cells as a longstanding 'mature' product will probably have an identifiable historical demand trend.

Is the present supply of product adequate or is there a demand gap? If there is a gap the size of this gap needs to be assessed and production planning altered to address this to achieve adequate supply at current levels. This of course assumes that the funding resources and donors are available for this to be achieved.

What is the likely increase in this demand in the planning period? This will either be the increase from current supply levels or the increase that will occur once any current gap is partially or completely filled.

What impacts could potentially also impact demand, taking it away from what would otherwise be the demand increase or decrease driven by current factors? These include a range of important factors any one of which may have a sizeable impact

- a change in clinical practice or indications
- demographic changes
- the introduction of new or alternative products
- improvements in inventory practice
- decreases in wastage and expiry
- autologous blood

To take each of these in turn

Never underestimate the value of assessing the historical demand for the product. Assessing some of the other factors below may be very difficult and at the end of the day the historical trend may be just about the most concrete and reliable predictor of demand. It is after all a measure of something real, something that has actually happened. It is free of all the uncertainty of predicted changes and what could happen. Its weakness of course is that it is historical. In my experience the more consistent the historical trend has been the more reliable it is likely to be as an indicator of future demand. Furthermore, the greater the change or impact that will be required to change that trend. In most instances red cells as a high volume, 'mature' product will have an identifiable and clear historical trend. For Australia this trend has been around 1%. Thus the historical demand trend will act as a logical starting point to be adjusted as appropriate by assessments of other relevant factors.

A change in clinical practice or indications could perhaps be best exampled by a change in the transfusion trigger or haemoglobin threshold. A move by users from the more historical setting of 10 g/dl to a level of 8g/dl will have a potential impact on the requirement for red cells. In Australia as in other developed countries there has been such a move with the introduction of national guidelines representing best practice [9]. The UK has also introduced a comprehensive approach to the better management of blood and the changing indications for red cell use in the north of England have also recently been reviewed [10,11].

Demographic changes aside from general population increases will also need to be considered. An example of the impact of demographic changes has recently been provided by a German study [12]. Demographic changes are interesting in that whilst they only have very gradual impact overtime from a total population perspective they actually create sudden jumps in demand. This is because the health infrastructure will not usually be able to seamlessly change over time to match the demographic change. Instead what happens is that a new hospital, or ward or treatment unit will open as a piece of new infrastructure.

The introduction of new or alternative products whilst appearing unlikely in the short term could have very significant future impacts. A recent innovation of the introduction of malarial testing in Australia is increasing the number of usable red cells and is an example of how new technology can impact production planning [13]. The successful introduction of blood substitutes would dramatically affect the demand for whole blood red cells and of course plasma volume expanders including albumin products [14]. The increased use of erythropoietin may also have an impact in the medium to long term [15].

Autologous blood may or may not also play a significant role in a blood system. Its use varies internationally by country and by regulation. Whatever its role, it must be taken into account in the planning process. Studies of autologous blood collections in Canada and Germany have recently been published [16,17]. Patient and public interest has also recently been surveyed [18,19].

Improvements in inventory practice again may well impact on demand by ensuring lower stock requirements through moves to type and screen practices and electronic cross matching. Improvements in stock rotation will also be a factor. The ability to centralise stock holdings through increased cooperation and improved transport and distribution systems will also play a potential role.

Decreases in wastage and expiry are sadly required in many health systems. On the bright side this creates the opportunity to ease the burden on supply whilst at the same time ensuring that the donor's precious gift is used. Whilst we might assume it, and our donors expect it, unaudited user groups will almost certainly have some unnecessary wastage. This will not be limited to on-the-shelf expiry of red cells but also the waste resulting from technical and mechanical problems such as fridge and alarm failures.

The Australian Red Cross Blood Service (ARCBS) in Australia has recently found red cell discard rates ranged from <1% to 6.5% for metropolitan hospitals, and up to 28% for regional/remote organisations [20].

The final factor to be taken into account is the breakdown of demand by ABO Rh groups. Generally in western countries and certainly in Australia there is a disproportionately high demand for O Negative red cells. Equally there is a disproportionately low demand for group AB red cells. Consequently most transfusion services constantly have low levels of O Negative red cells but high levels and wastage rates of AB product. Note that this does not mean that expiry rates of O Negative red cells by hospitals should assumed to be low. In fact the reverse is often the case, particularly in smaller more geographically remote hospitals where O Negative red cells may be kept for emergencies. These emergencies may in fact have very low probabilities of occurring and in my experience common sense negotiation with these institutions can be a very fertile way of improving the efficiency of use of this most precious resource. As already described above ARCBS found the discard rate for O- red cells was four times the rate for O+ and twice the rate for A [20].

The practice of providing red cell units matched for groups other than ABO and Rh, for example Kell, in situations other than where antibodies exist has varied internationally and may or may not need to be assessed as part of the demand equation. An internal forum has looked at this practice [21].

The Particular Problem of Platelets

Adequate national planning for the demand of platelets has been a longstanding challenge for blood bankers. The shelf life of platelets is currently limited to 5 or at most 7 days although one study suggests that aphaeresis platelets may be able to be stored for as long as 8 days [22]. This short shelf life creates a short term planning pressure in addition to the requirements of the annual production plan [23]. It is the constant demand for platelets that will ultimately be a major determinate of the opening hours of collection centres particularly whether they are open on weekends and public holidays.

Factors affecting platelet demand need to be assessed just as for red cells. The platelet trigger, particularly for prophylactic platelet transfusion, much debated over many years in the literature, is a key driver particularly if a change in practice occurs.

Holidays are difficult times for meeting platelet demand. Generally demand is difficult to predict and it will fluctuate significantly from year to year however the value of close liaison with the major platelet using hospitals regarding anticipated patient load, required groups and collaboration between centres holding inventory should not be underestimated.

The need for ABO group specificity is also a key factor to be considered. Historically with the use of random platelets derived from whole blood practice varied internationally with some countries always striving for ABO group compatibility while others, including the USA have had many users happy to transfuse across ABO group barriers. The advent of pooled and in particular aphaeresis platelets has increased the need for vigilance to avoid significant ABO haemolytic reactions. An international forum has reviewed the practice of transfusion of aphaeresis platelets and ABO groups [24].

Also critical is the agreed platelet transfusion trigger, dosing practices and the use and extent of adherence to any guidelines and whether there is likely to any significant change in these during the planning period [25-28].

Fresh Frozen Plasma

The use of clinical fresh frozen plasma varies considerably from country to country however one theme that appears all too often is that audits of clinical practice frequently demonstrate considerable inappropriate use of this product [29]. Wastage is also often a factor through both unnecessary expiry, non use of thawed units and breakage of frozen units due to the brittleness of the product [20]. ARCBS has found that 38% of discards were due to product being thawed and not subsequently used within the limited time specified. Further 25% of discards were due to damage to the fragile product. Again however, it is the potential for the change in demand that is as critical as anything else for the production planner and substantial changes in clinical behaviour following audit can occur [30,31].

Other Fresh Products

Other fresh products will generally be used in much lower volumes but each will need to be taken into account in the planning process especially where their manufacture is the result of further processing of one of the high volume products for example the manufacture of cryoprecipitate and /or cryosupernate from units of clinical fresh frozen plasma. Further examples of lower volume fresh products include washed and frozen red cells, pediatric products and highly phenotyped or CMV negative products.

PLASMA PRODUCT DEMAND

Introductory Note

The extent to which the planning for plasma products affects the production planner depends greatly on the role which they are going to play and in particular whether that role includes the collection of all or part of the plasma from which these products will be made. In an entirely open market as is the case in many parts of the world planning plasma product supply to meet national demand means ensuring that appropriate purchasing contracts are in place with manufacturers. These could be the responsibility of government agencies or the blood service itself. The issue of sourcing plasma in the context of fractionation and future plasma product demand has recently been extensively reviewed in the Australian context [32]. Where the national production planning extends to the procurement through collection of the starting plasma, the assessment of the demand itself will be important, but the responsibility for ensuring that it is able to be met may extend to those bodies responsible for funding.

Albumin

Historically the supply of albumin has been central to plasma product supply. However in the majority of developed countries and certainly in Australia the need for albumin is easily able to be met as it can be made from the same plasma as IVIG which is a key driver for plasma collection. In other words there will generally be more than enough plasma for albumin production, the main concern being how much albumin is actually required. The role of albumin versus saline has been a long debated issue relevant to the planner with significant fluctuations in demand internationally culminating in the SAFE trial [33].

Coagulation Factors

Factor VIII in Australia is illustrative of how fast things can change. Until the mid 1990's Australia had had shortages of factor VIII struggling to met the WHO target of the use of 2 units of Factor VIII per head of population. It had been the driver of the requirement for plasma for fractionation.

From the mid 1990s two significant changes meant that the driving role of Factor VIII began to change. First there was the gradual appearance of recombinant factor VIII products albeit under restricted usage criteria. In addition the demand for intravenous immunoglobulin meant that it was in even shorter supply than factor VIII and it rapidly became the overall driver of plasma production as it remains today.

Since 2000 two further changes have continued plasma derived factor VIII on its see sawing ride of supply and demand balance. The decision by Government in Australia to make recombinant factors available to patients as preferred products meant that suddenly there was for the first time a huge surplus of production capacity for plasma derived Factor VIII of some 40million units as it now made up only some 15% of demand. However just when it seemed that its days as a plasma driver had finally ended new criteria for vCJD donor deferral meant that only 30% or of the previously available plasma could now be used for plasma derived Factor VIII production and just as quickly as the potential surplus appeared it had gone again! At the time of writing it seems that the situation has yet again reversed.

Estimates of future demand of the plasma derived product in Australia are hard to predict, such is the lot of a production planner! Something as simple as a further review of a policy or product approval could, and it seems probably has, once again put Australia back into the position of significant surplus production capacity. Australia recently developed forecasts for all the required plasma products as part of the Review of Australia's Plasma Fractionation Arrangements [32].

Immunoglobulins

Traditionally three are broad immunoglobulin product types, intravenous immunoglobulin (IVIG), normal immunoglobulin (both the traditional intramuscular products and the new subcutaneous products) and specific hyperimmune immunoglobulins. This is relevant as although IVIG will be the main plasma driver only one the three broader product types can be manufactured from any given litre of plasma. Thus crucially the total amount of plasma required for fractionation will be the amount required for the quantity needed for these three product ranges added together. Thus as a consequence, accurate determination of demand for all three of these immunoglobulins is important in the planning process.

Others

Many other plasma products can be made from fractionated plasma. In the main these can be manufactured from starting plasma in addition to immunoglobulins. Each service must determine both the demand and need for these. Examples include anti-thrombin III, C-1-esterase inhibitor, alpha 1 anti-trypsin and others however a detailed analysis of these products is beyond the overall scope and detail of the current chapter.

Production of Products

Fresh Products

Generally the drivers will be either red cells or platelets or both. The extent to which the production of these is interlinked is dependent on the method of platelet production. The traditional method of production of platelets from platelet rich plasma means that there was a strong linkage to red cell product and in extreme circumstances was the driver of the collection of whole blood. Buffy coat pooled platelet production retains this link while the manufacture of part or all of the platelet supply through aphaeresis creates a dual production line with the aphaeresis platelet production impacting and perhaps adding to the amount of plasma being generated particularly for fractionation.

In calculating the production requirements for each fresh product not only will the demand and any change it undergoes be important but also the internal losses that will occur due to the need to sustain inventory requirements in multiple locations, expiry and losses due to unusable units, for example any units manufactured from donors who have been to a malarious area.

Plasma Products

In one sense this is a simple matter as plasma product manufacture is a highly specialist pharmaceutical activity carried out by increasingly by a relatively small number of large global players who may also procure their own starting plasma. For those planners who are also responsible for the procurement of the starting plasma involved it can be a more challenging exercise.

A plasma model will need to be developed taking into account whichever of the immunoglobulin types required. The ARCBS in Australia requires plasma to generate a range of immunoglobulins that are mutually exclusive in terms of their plasma source. Whilst intravenous immunoglobulin and intramuscular normal immunoglobulin can be made from the same plasma, only one or the other can be made. Hyperimmune globulins can only be made from plasma with adequate levels of the specific antibody relevant to the product being made. Thus in this sense the plasma required for each of these products is additive with the additional caveat that the plasma for the hyperimmunes must meet particular antibody specificity requirements.

Yield is the crucial determinant of the amount of plasma required and is generally available and straightforward all products except the hyperimmunglobulins. Difficulty exists with yields for hyperimmune immunoglobulins as the quantity or titer of antibody in the starting plasma is important and often varies considerably between batches. In fact for a product such as Rh D immunoglobulin the yield in any given batch can be determined by the presence or absence of a single high level antibody donor. Countries must decide whether the collection of these special and specific plasmas will be part of their own national program or whether it is easier and more economic to simply purchase manufactured product in the international market.

Once the demand of the products are known and the yield ascertained then the amount of starting plasma to be fractionated can be ascertained and in turn the product or products that will be the drivers of the overall quantity of plasma can be determined. For most developed countries that have largely moved to recombinant Factor VIII and IX products the current driver will be Intravenous immunoglobulin (IVIG) although as already discussed above this can change with a single policy change!

Once the drivers are determined then the overall quantities of plasma of various types can be worked out. If IVIG is the driver (as opposed to Factor VIII or albumin) then the overall plasma required will be that required for the IVIG plus that required for any normal immunoglobulin production plus that required for any hyperimmunglobulin production.

The Annual Cycle within the Plan

Is demand going to be even across the year? This is an important question as seasonal variations for products may vary considerably especially for fresh products. In Australia there is quite a strong cycle reflected in red cell stocks meaning that there is generally a fall in red cell stocks after the Easter break leading into the winter months with shortages often experienced around May/June and again in August/September. Each country will have its own cycles driven by its own circumstances including climate and holiday periods together with hospital activity.

The Need for Inventory

Inventory will be needed for all products. If you have a shortage of any particular product now inventories will be low or very low unless there is an alternative product being sourced or, undesirably, issues are being constrained for the purpose of building an inventory. In future planning for product supplies the need to build inventory in addition to matching changes in demand may be as big or even greater challenge as the demand itself. Whatever the difficulties they will need to be factored in. Equally to expect to build inventory of a product which is in overall short supply is probably unrealistic as a short term goal.

The inventory challenges will also vary considerably between products. The inventory challenges of platelets with a five day expiry are different to red cells with a 42 day expiry which are different again to plasma products which may have a shelf life of several years.

Routine versus exceptional demand also needs to be taken into consideration. In the main inventory will need as a minimum to be able to withstand the inevitable fluctuations associated with everyday usage by a health system. No two days may be same nor should they be expected to be. A more difficult issue is how to cope with significant surges in demand for example in the case of products needed in disasters or the sudden outbreak of conflict. For products in short expiry it is difficult, and in my view it is not sensible to carry large inventories with consequent wastage through expiry for the "what if" scenarios which rarely occur. Some further aspects of this are discussed under Shortages below.

For plasma products the situation is more difficult as large quantities can't be manufactured overnight. The important thing with these products is to have assessed what may be needed in various types of situations. Albumin in conflict situations is an obvious example but the sudden need for large quantities of normal immunoglobulin in a Hepatitis A outbreak in an exposed, unvaccinated population with low levels of natural immunity can also present significant challenge. Australia has managed these types of problems through the creation of national reserves of plasma products. Here product levels are built up to an agreed target level with quantities of newly manufactured products rotated into the reserve to replace short expiry product which is rotated out for general use to prevent unnecessary large scale expiry.

Surplus Products

The mere fact that one or more products will be the drivers of production means that there will be others that are not and for which there will be excess production capacity. This is most relevant for plasma products where IVIG as a driver can lead to considerable excess capacity to produce both albumin and factor VIII. Some other plasma products may have a considerable production capacity excess regardless of the plasma product driver. Examples may include plasma derived factor IX and antithrombin III concentrates.

In other cases a country may simply have an ability to manufacture more than it needs, even of fresh products. An example here is the former Euroblood Program which started in 1973 and ended in 2002 involving the shipment of red cells from Europe to the USA [34]. At its peak it made up some one third of the red cell supply to the New York area [35]. As a minimum there must be a system for surpluses of product to be moved from region to region within the national framework. Examples for reference can be sourced from the UK and the AABB in the US [1,36].

There are some interesting and perhaps challenging ethical and economic issues that arise in discussing surplus products. However perhaps the most important point to be considered up front is whether the surplus has arisen unexpectedly or deliberately, and whether it is likely or able to be ongoing.

Ethically it would seem that for surplus manufactured product to expire unused in any sizable quantity anywhere at any time is not only poor planning but also a lost opportunity for others less fortunate to be helped. The decision not to use the ability to make surplus product is a more complicated problem. This has been shown with the introduction of recombinant factor VIII and the ability not always utilised for large quantities of plasma derived product to be generated and the Canadian experience in moving to recombinant Factor VIII is illustrative [37,38].

Economics also plays a role in two ways. First there is a cost in the manufacture of any product and the deliberate manufacture of a surplus means that a cost will knowingly be incurred. How will that cost be met? Will the product supply be paid for through direct payment or an aid process with or without Government backing? If no payment is likely, it would seem unreasonable for a manufacturer to deliberately generate large surpluses of anything.

The other way that the economic question can be framed is that the sale of surplus product is potentially a way for a producer to subsidise the manufacture of existing products or the development and introduction of new ones. The Norwegian plasma fractionation project is a good case study [39].

There are numerous potential barriers that will probably need to be overcome in surplus product movements. These will frequently include legislative, regulatory, political, commercial interests, public perception and others. However none of these should be insurmountable if there is the will and the case is strong.

Why Wastage is so Important and Unnecessary!

It can be argued that provided there is no dramatic change to wastage levels it is a 'constant' that is of minimal impact to a production planner however I take a different view. Unnecessary and avoidable wastage is unacceptable and must be identified and forthrightly addressed. If for no other reason this is because the production planner will have to produce fewer products to meet the same demand. However the reasons are more significant than this. How can anyone justify any wastage of donations to their blood donors, especially those who are voluntary and unremunerated? How can it be ethical to go to the public and appeal for blood to overcome shortages when there is avoidable waste of what is already available?

Wastage of course comes in a number of forms. On the shelf expiry is of course one of the significant ones. No one would argue that some on the shelf expiry is unavoidable. However this can and should be minimised. It will vary between products and generally it is particularly difficult for platelets.

Other forms of wastage must also be recognised and controlled. Product failure is an issue of quality control and assurance. Transport and storage failures also can potentially add up to greater losses than might generally be recognised. Product transported out of storage temperature, through time delays, being left in trucks, railway stations or airport tarmacs should be completely avoidable. Refrigeration failures in facilities, either suppliers or hospitals are frustrating and again avoidable. Facilities known to have non compliant storage equipment or a track record of significant product loss should not be storing product until definitive evidence of correction of their problems is documented. Facilities that have compliant equipment but fail to save product in case of equipment failure either have no backup facility to move the product to or all too often have a failure of action due to inability to contact the staff who would be able to take action. These problems are particularly common in out of hours failures and can unfortunately occur in facilities holding significant amounts of product.

Shortages

The risk and consequences of shortages are what makes the management of production planning the crucial task that it is! While the total annual plan is the basic platform it is necessary to ensure that there is sufficient of all products all the time. Most services will have predictable times of the year where demand will be higher or lower than the overall average as discussed earlier and this must be factored into the planning process.

On the other hand shortages can also occur anytime due to sudden and unpredictable demand for product. These shortages when impacting fresh products can often be ABO group specific. These need to be overcome with good donor recruitment strategies but can be challenging if repeated appeals are made to the public with almost a 'crying wolf' situation at risk of developing.

The one perceived cause of shortage that rarely needs specific action is a disaster situation. In these situations two factors act to make a real shortage of product a rare event indeed. Firstly and tragically large scale disasters frequently have a much lower need for product than is often assumed as the fatality rate is high. The second is that the human spirit and desire to help ones fellow man creates an often unstoppable surge of willing donors who may queue for hours to donate. In these situations there may be a greater need to turn donors away than to encourage more to come forward. In my experience and others, for example the 911 disaster, the greater problem may be the management of a sudden massive stock, for example of red cells, without an immediate need for their use and the limited 42 day expiry [40]. Suggestions have been made to solve this dilemma of this situation through large scale freezing of red cell units but the cost and facility requirements make this largely impractical. The impact of red cell freezing on the supply chain has been reviewed [41]. Shortages can occur in plasma products as well. A Canadian study has looked at the changes in IVIG prescribing patterns in a period of shortage [42].

Disaster planning has recently taken on a new level of importance with the need to consider the management of disasters that have a major impact on the donor population as well as the need for blood and blood products. The prototype for this scenario has been the planning for the management of a flu pandemic following concerns of the impact of the H5N1 bird flu strain. Detailed disaster scenario planning is beyond the scope of this chapter but readers are directed to recent publications of national planning in this area [43,44].

The Plenty Paradox

The greater the supply of product, the greater the wastage generally is through expiry. To some extent this is unavoidable and very high stock levels may simply mean that more has been collected than could ever be used. The paradox however is that it is at high stock levels rather than situations of shortage where inventory practice can become an important tool to avoid large amounts of wastage at the very time when everyone has less reason to worry about it. There is less incentive for hospitals to maximize the utlisation of products through optimised inventory practices. A second issue is that when the blood supply facility has high inventories it will tend to issue stock with shorter expiry to hospitals giving them less time to utilise the products. This second problem is a bigger issue when product, for example red cells, is issued to hospitals with a high coefficient of variation of usage and studies looking at the age of red cell units at the time of transfusion are also of interest on this point [45,46].

At low stock levels people will be doing everything they can to get hold of and use every unit or bottle of product in shortage! At levels where supply is good but not necessarily above the demand, expiry may still be at higher than desired levels.

A Hypothetical National Model

So how does all this translate into the production plan itself? There are doubtless many ways to look at building this however a logical process that could be followed is suggested below. Let us suppose that the following hypothetical requirements exist for a country with a population of 10 million people that has red cells (required at a rate of 35 per 1,000 population) as its fresh product demand driver and IVIG (required at a rate of 70g per 1,000 population) as its plasma product demand driver with a national policy of plasma product self-sufficiency all collected by its national blood service.

In addition to the red cells (non-leucodepleted or leucodepleted, washed, frozen etc) it has additional fresh product requirements for platelets, clinical FFP, cryoprecipitate and some other low volume products others including whole blood, washed red cells and a frozen red cell phenotyped rare red cell bank. It also has plasma product requirements for albumin, plasma derived Factor VIII, plasma derived factor IX, normal immunoglobulin and tetanus and zoster immunoglobulins. It sources all other specific hyperimmune globulins on the international commercial market.

Thus as the red cell driver 350,000 units of red cells will be required to be supplied to meet the demand. If there is an internal red cell expiry of 1% within the blood service then to have 350,000 red cells issued there will be an annual requirement to produce 353,534 issuable red cells. To then work out how many red cell units need to be manufactured to achieve this one then needs to upscale this figure to take into account the manufacture of any red cell units that are manufactured but are unable to be used for whatever reason. Let us say that for various reasons (eg malarial risk) 5% of all whole blood donations collected are unable to have transfusable red cell units made from them. This means that 353,534 red cells must in broad terms be 95% of the total whole blood units (donations) collected. This gives us a figure of 372,141 whole blood donations. To this must finally be added any requirement for units of whole blood (which should be very low in a modern blood supply) and any special red cell products for example red cell panels. If we say for ease of calculation this takes us up to a round figure of some 375,000 donations to service this population at the required red cell transfusion rate.

Once the number of red cell units to be produced is known then the total quantity of recovered plasma from those original whole blood units that should be available for fractionation can be estimated. We do this by taking the estimated number of plasma units and taking away those that will be required for clinical fresh frozen plasma and cryoprecipitate/cryosupernate production. If we say that we can generate some 375,000 300ml recovered plasma units and there is a requirement for 50,000 units of clinical FFP and 20,000 units of cryoprecipitate (assuming more cryoprecipitate is needed than cryosupernate) then there should be some 305,000 300ml recovered plasma units available for fractionation which is around 91,500 kg. From here the additional amount of plasma that will need to sourced by aphaeresis (with or without simultaneous platelet collection) can be estimated to ensure that the amount of IVIG required as the plasma driver can be generated together with the mutually exclusive requirements for normal and hyperimmune immunoglobulins.

So how much plasma will be required? To estimate this the yields of the immunoglobulin products in the fractionation process need to be known. As the driver the fractionator's yield for IVIg will be the most important of these. The IVIG yield will be determined by the efficiency of the processing technique used and the concentration of immunoglobulin in the starting plasma. This later will be impacted by the type of plasma (source plasma has lower immunoglobulin levels than recovered plasma) and the location as donor pools with exposure to multiple infectious agents, for example in tropical areas, will increase the yield. Thus it is important to know what the fractionator's yield will be from the plasma that you send as opposed to plasma from another source.

International IVIG yields are generally quoted as ranging from 3.5 to 5.5g per litre of plasma. For simplicity let us assume the fractionator will obtain a yield of 4.0g per litre of plasma. In our hypothetical case we need 700kg of IVIG to serve our population. At a yield of 4g per litre of plasma the 91500 kg of recovered plasma will generate 366 kg of the 700 kg required. Thus another 344 kg of product needs to be gained from source plasma (or all or part from imported product). If it is to be achieved through a self sufficient plasma model and the plasma yield for source plasma is also 4g per kg then a total of 86,000 kg needs to be generated by an aphaeresis program. One can easily see the challenge in this and equally the difficulty created in having products such as clinical FFP misused or wasted. Not only do the patients get a product they don't need it makes life much harder than it needs to be at the production end!

The number of donors required to generate this will depend on the volume of plasma collected at each donation and the frequency of donation of each individual donor. Note that some countries have policies on the amount of plasma that can be taken in a year from any one donor for example the Council of Europe [47]. The effects of intensive plasmapheresis on donors must be considered as part of the planning process. The long term effects of intensive plasmapheresis have recently been reported from a significant program [48].

To this plasma volume the volumes required for normal immunoglobulin and any hyperimmunes needs to be added. The calculation of the plasma volume requirement for normal immunoglobulin will be able to be based on an identifiable yield as the level of antibody in the overall donor pool will remain relatively constant. However even for this product caution needs to be taken. An example is if there is a requirement for minimum levels of some particular antibodies these may vary between plasma pools and over time. A recent example of importance in Australia has been the levels of Hepatitis A antibody. There have been improvements in hygiene and a decrease in natural infection and consequent immunity and more recently increased uptake of Hepatitis A vaccination. This has meant lower levels Hepatitis A antibody in pools of starting plasma making it more difficult to meet the level required in the product specification. This is able to be overcome with careful donor recruitment and planning, for example targeting older donors for manufacture of this particular product. However, the message is clear-planning is the key.

Hyperimmune immunoglobulin production presents specific problems to planners. In our hypothetical case our country needs tetanus and zoster immunoglobulin. The former will require recruitment of donors who have been immunized /boosted and have antibody levels above a level determined between the collection agency and the fractionator of the plasma into the final product. In a large scale program this will be able to be achieved and the average antibody level across the donor pool will have some predictability over time. Recruitment of donors and the predictability of antibody levels will be much more difficult for zoster immunoglobulin production. High levels will generally only be found in donors following recent occurrences of either chicken pox or shingles. Antibody levels will rapidly rise but then fall over a period of time meaning that these donors will have a limited time as contributors to the donor pool and new donors must be constantly sought.

Donor Planning

Having determined the production requirements for products the final step is to translate this into donor attendances in terms of both whole blood and aphaeresis. While beyond the scope of this chapter if it is not done well and the donors are not there when and where you need them all of the above planning will probably fail in achieving the overall objectives. Key questions that are part of this last but crucial step include the following.

How many donations in total will be required? How many of each type will be required?

Will demand be even across the year? Will donors be equally available through out the year? Answers to these questions will be the foundation of ultimate success.

Funding, Lead Time and the Planning Cycle

All of these could be a waste of time or at least merely serve to put funders on notice if funding is limited and unable to support the true demand. In systems where transfer pricing applies hospitals and clinicians and ultimately patients may be unable or unwilling to pay the costs of products even if they may clearly be of clinical benefit.

In systems where the blood provider is paid by government either as a budget or through a product unit price (PUP) such as in Australia, funders may be unable or unwilling to pay the costs of products even if they may clearly be of clinical benefit. Whatever the system the case for funding by whatever mechanism will need to be well reasoned and able to considered on an equal basis with all the other competing priorities that modern health systems face.

Conclusion

An adequate blood supply is one of the cornerstones of any health system. However it doesn't just happen and sound planning is the crucial step that must precede all other endeavours. Knowing current and future product needs enables this planning to be done on a sound basis. Anticipating trends and shifts in demand caused not only by increased usage but also improvements in managing wastage through decreased expiry and unnecessary transfusion will greatly assist the process. New products and changes in indications are also important as are adequate inventory levels. Finally the ability to find the donors and present sound cases for funding in a world of competing priorities is the glue that will ultimately enable the planning jigsaw to form the picture that we all want to see - a world where anybody can get the right product, at the right time, wherever they may be, every time!

REFERENCES

[1] Chapman J. F and Cook R. The Blood Stocks Management Scheme, a partnership between the National Blood Service of England and North Wales and participating hospitals for maximising blood supply chain management. *Vox Sanguinis* (2002) 83,239-246.

[2] Currie CJ, Patel TC, McEwan P, Dixon S. Evaluation of the future supply and demand for blood products in the United Kingdom. *Transfusion Medicine* (2004)14, 19-24.

[3] Ness P. M and Schiff P. Data collection: An unmet community transfusion need. *Transfusion* (2007) 47,373.

[4] Sazama K. The Ethics of Blood Management. *Vox Sanguinis* (2007) 92, 95-102.

[5] Leikola J. *Formulation of a national blood programme in Management of Blood Transfusion Services*, editor Hollan S. R (1990) WHO ISBN 92 4 154405 6.

[6] Leikola J. and Towle W. J. How Much Blood for the World? *Proceedings of the 19th Congress of the International Society of Blood Transfusion* (1986),Sydney

[7] Szilassy C. *Calculation of Present and Projected Blood Needs in Management of Blood Transfusion Services*, editor Hollan S. R (1990) WHO ISBN 92 4 154405 6.

[8] Cobain T. J. et al. A Survey of the Demographics of Blood Use. *Transfusion Medicine* (2007) 17, 1, 1-15.

[9] NHMRC Clinical Practice Guidelines for the use of Blood Components. (2001). Available from http://www. nhmrc. gov. au/publications/synopses/cp77syn. htm.

[10]Department of Health. Health Service Circular on *Better Blood Transfusion*: *Appropriate Use of Blood.* HSC 2002/009. (2002) Available at http://www. dh. gov. uk/en/PublicationsAndStatistics/LettersAndCirculars/HealthServiceCirculars/DH_4004264.

[11]Wallis J. P., Wells A. W. and Chapman C. E Changing Indications for red cell transfusion 2000 to 2004 in the north of England. *Transfusion Medicine* (2006) 16, 411-417.

[12]Greinacher A et al. Impact of demographic changes on the blood supply: Mecklenburg-West Pomerania as a model region for Europe. *Transfusion* (2007) 47,395-401.

[13]Seed C. R et al. The efficacy of a malarial antibody enzyme immunoassay for establishing the reinstatement status of blood donors potentially exposed to malaria. *Vox Sanguinis* (2005) 88, 98-106.

[14]Winslow R. M. The Current Status of Blood Substitutes. *Vox Sanguinis* (2006) 91,2, 102-110.

[15]Laird J. Erythropoietin: Can we afford to use it? Can we afford not to? *Transfusion Medicine* (2006) 16,204-205.

[16]Rock G. et al A review of nearly two decades in an autologous blood programme: the rise and fall of activity. *Transfusion Medicine* (2006) 16, 307-311.

[17]Kaufmann et al. A survey of autologous blood collection practices in Germany. *Transfusion Medicine* (2004) 14,335-341.
[18]Moxey A. J et al. Blood transfusion and autologous donation: a survey of post-surgical patients, interest group members and the public. *Transfusion Medicine* (2005) 15, 19-32.
[19]Banning M et al. Current perceptions of Canadian autologous blood donors. *Vox Sanguinis* (2006) 91,157-161.
[20]ARCBS Medilink December (2006). Available from http://www. transfusion. com. au/NEWS/Medilink. asp.
[21]International Forum. Red cell transfusions and blood groups. *Vox Sanguinis* (2004) 87,210-222.
[22]Slichter S. J et al. Viability and function of 8-day-stored aphaeresis platelets. *Transfusion* (2006) 46, 1763-1769.
[23]Pearson H et al Logistics of Platelet Concentrates. *Vox Sanguinis* (2007) 92, 160-181.
[24]International Forum. Transfusion of aphaeresis platelets and ABO groups. *Vox Sanguinis* (2005) 88,207-221.
[25]Heal J. M, Blumberg N. Optimizing platelet transfusion therapy. *Blood Reviews* (2004)18,149-65.
[26]Guidelines for the use of platelet transfusions. *Br J Haematology* (2003) 122, 10-23.
[27]Brecher M. E, Hom E. G, Hersh J. K. Optimal platelet dosing. *Transfusion* (1999) 39,431-432.
[28]Brecher M. E. The platelet prophylactic transfusion trigger: when expectations meet reality. *Transfusion* (2007) 47,188-191.
[29]Palo R et al. Population-based audit of fresh-frozen plasma transfusion practices. *Transfusion* (2006) 46, 1921-1925.
[30]Kakkar N, Kaur R and Dhanoa J. Improvement in fresh frozen plasma transfusion practice: results of an outcome audit. *Transfusion Medicine* (2004) 14,231-235.
[31]Yeh C. J et al Transfusion audit of fresh frozen plasma use in southern Taiwan. *Vox Sanguinis* (2006) 91,270-274.
[32]Flood P, Wills P, Lawler P, Ryan G, Rickard KA. Review of Australia's Plasma Fractionation Arrangements. (2006). Available from http://www. health. gov. au/plasmafractionationreview.
[33]Finfer S. A Comparison of Albumin in Saline for Fluid Resuscitation in the Intensive Care Unit. *New England Journal of Medicine* (2004) 350, 2247-2256.
[34]Morrell A. Alfred Hässig 1921–1999. *Vox Sanguinis* (2000) 78, 69-73.
[35]Center for Infectious Disease Research & Policy (CIDRAP), FDA panel favors new BSE-related rule on blood donations. (2005) available at http://www. cidrap. umn. edu/cidrap/content/other/bse/news/feb0905blood. html.
[36]Parham S. NBE Offers New "Spin" On Blood Resource Sharing AABB (2006) Available at www. aabb. org/documents/Programs_and_Services/National_Blood_Exchange/ nbex changenews06. pdf.
[37]Sher G. Canadian Blood Services. WFH Global Forum (2005) available at http://www. wfh. org/2/docs/Events/GF_14h15_Sher. ppt#256,1, *Canadian Blood Services.*
[38]Farrugia A. Safety and supply of haemophilia products: worldwide perspectives (2004) *Haemophilia* 10,327.

[39]Flesland O. Seghatchian J, Solheim B. G The Norwegian plasma fractionation project- a 12 year clinical and economic success story (2003) *Transfusion and Apheresis Science* 28, 93-100.

[40]Standley J. 'Waste' of 11 September donations. BBC (2002) available at http://news. bbc. co. uk/2/hi/americas/1833276. stm.

[41]Hess J. R, Red cell freezing and its impact on the supply chain. *Transfusion Medicine* (2004)14, 1-8.

[42]Pendergrast J. M, Sher G. D and Callum J. L. Changes in intravenous immunoglobulin prescribing patterns during a period of severe product shortages,1995–2000. *Vox Sanguinis* (2005) 89,150-160.

[43]Bedford R. Pandemic Influenza and the Blood Supply. UK Blood Services Emergency Planning Group. Available at_www. transfusionguidelines. org. uk/docs/pdfs/general_ pandemic-flu. pdf.

[44]WHO. Maintaining a Safe and Adequate Blood Supply in the Event of Pandemic Influenza (2006). Available at http://www. who. int/csr/disease/avian_influenza /guidelines/ bloodsupply/en/index. html.

[45]Pereira A. Blood inventory management in the type and screen era. *Vox Sanguinis* (2005) 89,245-250.

[46]Raat N. J. H et al. The age of stored red blood cell concentrates at the time of transfusion. *Transfusion Medicine* (2005) 15,419-423.

[47]Council of Europe. *Guide to the preparation, use and quality assurance of blood components-12th Edition* (2006). Council of Europe Publishing.

[48]Schulzki T et al. A prospective multicentre study on the safety of long-term intensive plasmapheresis in donors (SIPLA). *Vox Sanguinis* (2006) 91,162-173.

In: Transfusion - Think About It
Editor: Trevor J. Cobain

ISBN 978-1-61668-969-8

Chapter 3

KNOWING YOUR DONORS
STRATEGIC PLANNING FOR EVIDENCE-BASED DONOR RECRUITMENT AND RETENTION PROGRAMMES

Sheila F. O'Brien
National Epidemiology and Surveillance, Canadian Blood Services, Canada.

ABSTRACT

This chapter describes strategic planning for an evidence based approach towards recruitment and retention practice. Within this context, evidence-based practice means planning recruitment initiatives based on the best data and research available, and involves developing the skills amongst recruitment staff to make their own independent assessment of data and scientific literature. A four step model of assessment, planning intervention and evaluation is described, with particular focus on the assessment-evaluation loop. Rigorous scientific evaluation of interventions becomes the basis for further assessment and planning. Two aspects of strategy are described. Initially, a strategy to develop an organizational culture which is able to fully utilize evidence to develop recruitment strategy must be planned and implemented. With this in place, strategic directions for recruitment and retention can be developed, based on thorough assessment of the evidence, which will guide the development of specific interventions. Based on scientific assessment that regularly examines the 'big picture', looking beyond short term gains, some groups of donors will be identified where much effort yields little gain, but for other groups a targeted approach may be more promising. An evidence-based programme will focus energy and resources into high-yield activities, will make use of scientific methodology to evaluate the effectiveness of these activities, and will provide the knowledge base for continuous improvement.

Introduction

Strategy is an approach to thinking, planning and decision making that requires managers at all levels of the organization to know 'how things are' yet to make decisions that support 'how things should be'. Traditionally, thinking around recruitment and retention has been reactionary. The focus has been on finding out how people feel about blood donation, and finding ways to appeal to those feelings or views. As well, more attention has been paid to "doing" than to studying donors or evaluating outcomes. This chapter will focus on an evidence based approach to recruitment and strategic planning to develop and utilize evidence-based decision making. Strong leadership will encourage managers and recruitment professionals to generate scientifically sound donor data and to use such data to plan and evaluate initiatives.

The strategic direction recommended in this chapter is one that challenges management to lead their organizations from a quasi-evidence based culture to one that is fully evidence based at all levels of the organization. Within this context, evidence-based practice means planning recruitment initiatives based on the best data and research available, and involves developing the skills amongst recruitment staff to make their own independent assessment of data and scientific literature. Strategy for evidence based practice will necessarily challenge conventional wisdom, and require management to change the environment, not simply react to it. This should de-emphasize short-term micro-thinking, and expending excessive energy in low-yield activities, and emphasize long-term macro-thinking identifying (potential) donor groups where the greatest gains are likely to be made. It should result in thinking outside-of-the-box. For example, based on an assessment of current evidence, one may decide that rather than designing recruitment initiatives that appeal to the community's concepts and beliefs about blood donation, it may be more appropriate to change the community's beliefs. This is more difficult, and will have less immediate results, but could improve recruitment in the long run.

Although the focus in this chapter is on strategy relating to donor recruitment and retention, evidence based culture is a mind set that cannot be switched on for recruitment and then switched off for other matters, and so to go down this path the whole organization needs to think along these lines. In particular, it is the people who actually recruit and retain donors that need to understand and embrace evidence-based decision making. It can be encouraged by senior management in concrete ways, such as by setting in place structures that will facilitate the availability of data and expertise, and actively encouraging their routine application to recruitment practice.

Recruitment vs. Retention

Providing a safe and sufficient blood supply is dependant first and foremost on recruiting and retaining a base of blood donors who are committed to blood donation and pose minimal risk of transmissible disease. Although recruitment and retention are often discussed together, they are not the same. Recruitment involves identifying people who have never donated blood and motivating them to make a first attempt. Retention involves donors who have been recruited, made a first donation, and must be encouraged to become regular donors. Although continued recruitment of new donors is essential to balance donor loss, or build the donor base, the majority of blood donations come from repeat donors. In fact, it is much more efficient to retain donors than to recruit new ones. Recruitment and retention should be considered as a continuum so that there is a sound strategy not only for getting people to come to the collection site for the first time, but also to encourage them to return and become committed life-time donors. For example, the message that donors receive that encourages them to donate initially should be consistent with the message they receive when they actually donate and when they are invited to return to donate. The factors influencing retention of such donors may be different from those influencing recruitment of first-time donors, although there is likely some overlap.

The Assessment – Evaluation Loop

Using a four step model of assessment, planning, implementation and evaluation, strategic planning for evidence-based recruitment/retention will be described. Perhaps because recruitment and retention are very practical areas of expertise, there is a tendency to devote most of the effort to the middle two phases – planning and implementation. In this chapter we will therefore devote most of the attention to assessment and evaluation. These two steps generate the information necessary for the other steps. The process beginning with assessment and ending with evaluation of what was planned and implemented forms a loop in which the evaluation becomes part of the knowledge in re-assessment allowing for the developing strategy to adapt. The chapter focuses on the role of the assessment – evaluation loop for ongoing development of recruitment and retention strategy, but special attention has been given to strategic planning to put this process into place.

Why Do People Donate Blood?

The starting point that will be useful for the assessment phase is an understanding of why people donate blood, what affects the decision to donate and what keeps or prevents people from continuing to donate. Planning relates back to this foundation of knowledge. It is important to be cognisant of not just what is known (or thought to be known) but also what is not known. In particular, this should be evaluated very carefully by each blood establishment because the specific circumstances, such as the donation process in place, the accessibility of collection sites, and attributes of the general population form complex dynamics, and what may be true in one blood center may not necessarily be generalised to other regions.

Stages of Donation Career

Piliavin and Callero [1] describe a donation career as being a process towards commitment with some sort of initial identification or positive feelings about being a blood donor before the first donation (often involving association with donor role models). The first donation experience is pivotal. That is to say, the donor's positive perceptions must out-weigh the negative, and the development from seeing oneself as a non-donor to being a blood donor occur over several subsequent donations (but only if the donor has enough positive motivation to return). The positive and negative motivators have the most impact over the early stage of the donation career, and negative motivators have a greater likelihood of influencing people not to continue donation, but as the change to self recognition of 'I am a blood donor' occurs, the donor may perceive more positives than negatives, and be much less likely to be deterred from donation by a negative experience.

Because the early stage of donation is the most critical for continuation, recruiters often place considerable effort in trying to encourage new donors to return. Indeed, a continuous influx of new donors is essential. However, the majority of blood donations are collected from a relatively small group of dedicated, long term, committed donors. These donors have proven themselves as reliable and have demonstrated their ability to meet the selection criteria, and as there will inevitably be a few negative donation experiences in a long donation career, they have also demonstrated themselves to be resilient to such experiences. Strategies that are built on maximising collections from this group tend to be more cost effective – and more successful.

Altruism

Altruism, a social value that promotes behaviour that has no benefit for the donor but benefits the recipient, is often reported to be a primary motivator for blood donation. That donors express altruistic views is frequently discussed [2] although how it actually fits in to the decision to donate and to continue to donate is less clear.

Many people who are not blood donors have altruistic beliefs. Part of the challenge in recruitment may be to find ways to make the connection in the minds of potential donors of blood donation as a way of expressing altruistic beliefs. Appealing to altruism as a recruitment strategy is frequently done, however the extent to which people can relate the act of donating blood with giving to their community needs further exploration.

External Motivation

External motivation such as encouragement from donor friends and relatives, peer pressure and requests from recruiters probably play a substantial role in the decision to donate for the first time. External pressure by itself may not be enough to develop committed donors as the donating behaviour is likely to stop as soon as the pressure stops, or as the donor becomes more resistant to it. However, if the external pressure is merely a push that moves the donor from inertia to action then it could lead to development of commitment. Hence broad spectrum pressure tactics are less likely to yield committed donors, but it is possible that more targeted approaches would be effective if groups of people with personal characteristics that make them good candidates for donors can be identified.

CONVENIENCE

Donors have described convenience as an important factor in whether or not they will donate at any given time. In a US study of donors who had stopped donating roughly one third reported that not having a convenient place to donate was an important reason for not returning to donate [3]. This was an important reason for both first time and repeat donors who had stopped donating, and for different racial and ethnic groups. Intuitively, if it is not possible, or highly impractical to get to a collection site, people will not be able to donate. However, it is unclear how much inconvenience of the collection site is a true barrier, and how much it is a perceived barrier or rationalizing.

INCENTIVES

Blood programs composed of entirely volunteer donors are considered to be safer because donors should have less motivation to be untruthful in screening. It is certainly plausible that providing too much benefit for donating might encourage individuals at high-risk to become donors, however token gifts of little monetary value may be more acceptable. In a US survey, about 20% of donors said that they would be motivated to donate if they received items of small value, particularly younger donors and first time donors [4]. In a more recent survey [5] donors who gave blood at a center that provided gifts as incentives were more likely to rate such incentives as important motivators. Likewise donors who received supplemental health screening test were more likely to rate this as important compared with donors who donated at a center that did not offer such screening. The reasons for this observation are not clear, but could represent a self-fulfilling prophecy in which a center that provides incentives recruits donors who value the incentives, whereas the others recruit donors for whom incentives are less important. Alternatively, perhaps donors who might donate for other reasons come to see themselves as motivated by such incentives simply because they receive them. Also, when people state their motivation in a survey questionnaire, this may not have put very much thought into it, and it may not always reflect the true motivation.

In a randomized controlled trial comparing the incentive of a free t-shirt to entice first time donors back to make a second donation, there was no significant increase in donor return rates [6]. The lack of effect of this incentive could reflect the inability of people in the survey studies to estimate what would or would not motivate them, or perhaps the T-shirt was not motivating (not a good incentive), or perhaps donors who originally donate without incentives are not motivated by their addition.

MULTICULTURAL ISSUES

The proportion on non-white donors has been increasing over time with a study from 1991 to 1996 showing changes in first time donors indicating more new donors from ethnic and non-white race and fewer white donors across the US [7]. Even so, these proportions indicate that these groups are still under-represented in the donor population. A key challenge for recruiters in many countries is understanding motivational factors of people from many different ethnic backgrounds, and finding innovative ways of appealing to such donors.

Application of Recruitment Literature

Published data on donor behaviour is valuable, but the findings may not always hold true for every blood center. Sometimes reports appear to be conflicting. In such cases careful examination of the methods used, and the study population often reveal possible sources for the apparent conflict. It often is not so much that a given study was poor, but more that studies are different. It is by comparing different research reports that are all different that leads to new insight.

The heart of developing an evidence based culture is in critical evaluation of research – both in the literature and that produced internally. Encouraging an ability amongst recruitment staff to identify both the strengths and the limitations of published research is *the* most important step. From this, the knowledge and critical evaluation skills to plan and evaluate their own recruitment or retention initiatives will be in place. Depending on the starting point, this may require quite a bit of effort, but it will be well worth the investment. As many recruitment staff have little or no research training, some guidance, and some formal means of ensuring that staff can demonstrate the necessary skills may be appropriate

Assessing Recruitment and Retention Potential

An essential building block for strategic thinking is a thorough assessment of how things are at the present, and what advantages and limitations currently exist. Having identified these, it will then be possible decide what is being done well that should be continued, what should be changed, and to prioritise these. Since obtaining precise and reliable information is sometimes difficult, it is important to weigh up fairly early in the assessment process how important particular information is, and to place the most effort where it is going to count the most. As will be described, all of the information that might be desirable will not be available. Sometimes a simpler estimate will suffice, but there may be other areas where the data is sufficiently important to warrant collecting it yourself.

The assessment should show not only who donates and who does not, but must also delve into why things are the way they are. It should achieve a clear picture of where the greatest gains are likely to be made, as well as where you may do well to 'cut your losses' and accept that much effort will likely continue to yield little gain. This will challenge the 'we have got to do *everything* we can to get *every* donor that we can' approach, but the evidence should be persuasive. Once areas to maximise and minimise have been identified, the specific recruitment strategies can be planned.

Donor Demographics

Operational donor data can provide a useful 'snap-shot' of donors, and allows comparison with the general population. Demographic profile may be influenced by recruitment strategies applied previously, by the locations of collection sites, convenience factors, knowledge of the need for blood donation, etc. In other words it should not be assumed from the existing demographic profile, that donors matching this profile are necessarily the best 'target group' for recruitment – only that the observed demographic variables describe people who are known to be donors. It may be (in fact, it is likely) that other demographic groups could be recruited with different approaches or different circumstances.

Tables showing the number and percent of donors by demographic groupings such as gender, age group, number of donations and donation status are a good starting point. These relatively simple data can generate questions that will lead to a better understanding of who your donors are. For example, if there are more younger first-time donors than amongst repeat donors, is it because more young donors are being recruited at the present time or have young donors been recruited for a long time, but have not been retained? Thus, demographic data can be used to describe who the donors are, and can also give insight into why they are who they are.

This type of analysis can be produced from most databases, even those not set up specifically for donor research. The database only needs to have the capacity to sort the data into the categories and time frames and produce totals. A database capable of advanced statistical modeling can answer more questions, but may take some time to develop. With well defined questions, considerable insight into donor behaviour can be gained from very simple analyses, and so development of an evidence based recruitment and retention program can proceed while new database solutions are under development.

Donor Return Rates

With a more statistically sophisticated set-up, other information can be gained. By using Cox proportional-hazards models, which consider the time between two events (in this case donation dates), and by using a large dataset of over 800,000 first-time donors, it was reported that the shorter the time between a donor's first two donations, the more likely the donor was to make a subsequent donation [8]. This could mean that encouraging more frequent donations can lead to increased donor commitment, but could also be influenced by accessibility of donation sites. Others have applied logistic regression methods to examine donor return patterns [9]. It raises questions about the use of mobile collection units particularly when they are infrequent. The ability to obtain this type of information from one's own donor database clearly has benefits. Firstly, to confirm that this observation can be applied to a particular donor population, and secondly, if strategies are being implemented to increase the return of donors it will be possible to see if it resulted in an increase in subsequent donations.

Enhanced Data Collection

In the above examples, possibilities from databases using data that most blood centres currently collect (although not necessarily in a form that lends itself to analysis) were discussed. It can be seen that operational data can be quite informative but it is not possible to 'know your donors' based solely on this data. In the discussion on donor motivation, for example, most of the information comes from additional data collection, such as from donor interviews or surveys. Collecting additional data is essential, but should be based on a rigorous 'needs assessment' because it is time consuming, sometimes costly and only a small proportion of interesting topics can be explored.

The Eligible Population

The donor selection criteria exclude many people who might be willing to donate. The criteria vary by country, of course, and sometimes by blood establishment within a country. The selection criteria are intended to ensure that blood donation is safe for the donor, and that the blood donation will be as safe as possible for the blood recipient. Clearly this is essential, but it has the effect of narrowing down the 'eligible population'.

No-one really knows exactly how many people are eligible to donate in a given population, but a method for estimation has been described [10]. Using various population statistics in the US to estimate the proportion of the general population that failed to meet age criteria, and that had certain health problems or risk behaviours that were more common reasons for deferral, they estimated that about 59% of the US population were eligible to donate. The estimate required numerous assumptions, and therefore has some inherent inaccuracy, and some deferral reasons are difficult to quantify. However, the estimate suggests that the donor selection criteria narrow down the eligible population substantially, and although there appear to be enough eligible people to meet the need, the donor exclusion criteria clearly make the recruiters role more challenging.

The donor selection criteria definitely place some limitations on the potential donor pool in the general population, and make recruitment of donors more challenging, but they likely do not restrict the eligible donors to the point that it is an impossible task. An assessment of the eligible population, which can be done for sub-groups and regions within the blood establishment's area, can assist with evaluating the utility of recruitment methods such as 'cold calling' and recruitment among groups likely to have high proportions of ineligibility. This is part of the assessment for deciding if a more targeted approach is needed, and what that approach should be.

Impact of Temporary Deferral

Permanent deferral criteria remove the donor from the potential donor pool altogether, and some temporary deferrals that donors may repeat regularly amount to permanent deferral. For example, some people travel to malaria risk areas frequently, and even though the deferral for malaria risk travel is a temporary deferral, the repetitive nature of such travel often makes donation rarely possible, or even impossible for such individuals.

Temporary deferral contributes considerably to donor ineligibility. In the US, a little under 10% of donors are deferred temporarily with short term deferral, with about 2.8% also deferred for longer term (such as malaria travel) [11]. The impact of deferral policy should not be seen as only impacting upon 'eligible' or 'not eligible'. Deferral policies may impact upon recruitment and particularly retention with donors less likely to return after temporary deferral. In the US, Custer et al [12] tracked donor return rates after temporary deferral and reported that donor return was lower for both first-time and repeat donors after being deferred compared with non-deferred donors. In another study in a US blood donors with deferrals for low hemoglobin, elevated blood pressure and abnormal pulse, which accounted for more than half of the temporary deferrals (46% were for low haemoglobin), were more likely to be deferred again if they returned [13]. Many such donors could be eligible some of the time, but it may be very 'hit and miss' whether they can donate at any given time. Hence, de-motivation after deferral is only part of the effect. Donors may also have reasonable doubt of being eligible if they do return.

Assessment weighing up the benefit of attempting to keep deferred donors coming back with the costs of doing so, such as appointment times that may not yield a donation, and the amount of effort and resources being used should be done. An important outcome of this is deciding whether it is worthwhile expending effort to encourage donors to return after deferral, and if so, which deferrals or demographic groups are good candidates for such effort.

Technological Support

An area of considerable interest among blood establishments is the innovative use of technology. Email is a very cost effective method of communicating, although not without some problems. The use of web sites for informing donors, helping donors to assess eligibility, and perhaps make appointments are potential aids to recruitment and retention that should be explored.

From Ongoing Assessment Strategy Develops

Based on the assessment, evidence-based recruitment strategy can be developed. Assessment of 'how things are' must stimulate thoughtful reflection on 'how things should be'. At this point in the process it is essential to avoid 'shooting-down' ideas simply because the logistics of getting there are not clear at the time.

In order to illustrate how the process should be used, consider some possibilities that might hypothetically arise from an assessment. Let's say that the assessment indicated that attempting to retain certain groups of deferred donors (or maybe deferred donors in general) was likely to be low-yield and high effort, and so you make a decision not to expend effort on this. Let's also say the average number of donations per donor is about 2 per year although they are eligible to donate about 5 times per year– 'how things are'. The assessment should explain why things are the way they are. For example, if half of the collections are from mobile units and many of them only come to an area once or twice a year, that will explain some of it. Examining the call center activities may give some indications as to whether people are generally unwilling to come in more than twice a year, or if they are just likely to only be asked twice a year. If some are unwilling, do you know why? Now you need to decide what the ideal donation rate should be – 'how things should be'. If the donation rate increased to 3 donations per year, this would increase collections by 50%, 4 donations per year would double it. Of course, more donations per donor, means more donations are lost per donor lost. Let's say you decide that an ideal donation rate is 3 donations per donor per year. The assessment has given some indications of what has held the donation rate at 2, and where changes are likely to have the greatest impact.

The strategy that is now emerging is one in which some low yield activities have been identified and discontinued, which frees up some energy and resources for focusing on higher yield initiatives. The assessment should have yielded some initial direction for retention initiatives, perhaps targeted call center activity, and it is now much clearer where to focus further assessment. In this way, interventions can be planned, with further assessment simultaneously (such as more detailed information about what might encourage people to donate more frequently), and along with the evaluation of the intervention, further interventions will be planned.

The above example is somewhat simplified to delineate the thinking behind the assessment evaluation loop, and a full assessment will include many factors. It is important, nevertheless, to distil the high yield and low yield areas down to no more than two or three of each in order to focus planning and implementation.

EVALUATION METHODS

This section discusses some of the possible tools that blood establishments can consider to evaluate the effectiveness of recruitment initiatives. The main pitfalls in evaluation are inferring too much from weak data, and not placing enough weight on stronger evidence. A variety of approaches is desirable, but each has advantages and disadvantages.

Data Gathering for the Evaluation-Assessment Loop

Obtaining information from different sources, using different methods is an advantage. Each approach has its advantages and disadvantages.

Qualitative Data

Focus Groups and Qualitative Interviews

In its broadest sense, this is information that cannot be condensed into numeric form, at least not easily. In-depth interviews with donors, and focus groups are often used to explore how people are thinking on different topics. It is often the first place to start when trying to understand something new. Although the detail and depth of information from qualitative methods is generally superior to that of surveys or donor databases, the information cannot be generalized to donors who were not interviewed. Qualitative research is used more extensively when preparing donor advertising or donor educational materials because the donor needs to view the materials and provide feedback. It is best used, therefore, as a starting point rather than a final evaluation.

Donor Feedback Methods

Donor feedback can be solicited in a variety of ways. Frequently a 'suggestion box' is located in the collection site for this purpose. Web-based feedback mechanisms can allow for similar data to be collected. In addition, donors sometimes telephone or write to the blood center with suggestions or concerns. These methods are good for donor relations and form an opportunity to stay in touch with donors. However, people often are more motivated by dissatisfaction than praise, so such methods tend to provide more information on what donors are not happy about or think should be improved, and provide less feedback on what is being done that donors like and want to see continued. Also, the views expressed in suggestion boxes are not necessarily representative of donors in general, so this form of feedback should stimulate thought, but should not form the basis for decision making.

Data Describing Donors - Donor Surveys

Donor surveys are an excellent way to gather donor information. If appropriate random donor selection methods are applied, and the donor response rate is at an acceptable level, donor surveys can provide information that is generalizable to the donor base. Donor surveys are key to data gathering for assessment in which one wishes to understand donor issues to plan recruitment and retention initiatives. As an evaluative tool, donor surveys can be conducted at time intervals to assess things such as change in attitudes or to see if recruitment initiatives were noticed by donors (eg advertising) and gain feedback on their views about it. Surveys can be targeted to specific groups of donors such as those who attended a collection site on a particular date or to a specific demographic profile. Interpretation of survey data can be difficult, since donor attitudes are influenced by many things and people have difficulty articulating what exactly has influenced their opinions, if they are conscious of this at all. In addition, as the outcome of greatest interest in evaluation of interventions is the actual effectiveness of the intervention, this is more concretely measured by actual donor behaviour (eg did they actually donate?).

Evaluating Recruitment/Retention Initiatives – Intervention Studies

The most concrete measurement of the effectiveness of an intervention is the number of donors who attend a collection site, and make a donation. However, simply counting the number of donations after an intervention and presuming there is a cause-effect relationship can be misleading because:

1) There is a certain amount of variation from one time period to another that is not related to anything that was done.

And

2) Sometimes other things that have occurred at the same time, either other recruitment initiatives done at the same time, or other independent events in the community may influence donations.

Methods for evaluating initiatives must control for these extraneous events in order to give meaningful results.

Depending upon the circumstances, a variety of evaluative methods could be useful. The following are some standard methods that will serve to highlight some of the important features of design, and some of the strengths and limitations to consider.

Randomised Controlled Trials

Randomised controlled trials (RCTs) provide the most air-tight level of evidence. One needs to be able to randomly assign donors to either the intervention group or the control group, and so a list of people is normally a prerequisite. For example, in a study designed to determine if sending a personalized letter that included information about the donor's blood type and about the percentage of the general population with the same blood type who donated would increase donor return rates in early-career donors, donors were stratified by blood group (rare, common or universal blood types) and randomly assigned to receive either this new letter (the experimental group) or a recruitment letter with some general information (the control group). Donors were then tracked to determine how many returned after the letter, and it was found that donors in the experimental letter were significantly more likely to return [14]. This design is very sound because the random assignment of donors to the groups controls for possible extraneous factors. By doing this, all other things are equal, including events in the community or other initiatives that the Center may have been doing at the same time. In addition the stratifying of donors by blood group ensured that the proportion of donors from each blood group was similar in the experimental and control groups which was an important part of this intervention, hence any impact of blood group was controlled for by the design. It is therefore reasonable to conclude that increased return rate observed was due to the receiving the experimental letter.

RCT's can be done with a number of variations. For example, a study by Reich et al [6] employed a two by two factorial design to their RCT in which two telephone messages (message 1 was routine, message 2 was novel) were compared, and the impact of an incentive (a free T shirt) was also studied. This resulted in 4 groups: message 1, no incentive, message 1 with incentive, message 2 no incentive and message 2 with incentive. With this design it was possible to determine if there were independent contributions of message 2 and the incentive, and if this was additive (that is, if there were more donors when both were received). The group that received message 1 and no incentive served as the control group. In their study message 2 was effective but the incentive was not.

RCT's are very sound methodologically, and are often seen as the 'gold standard' for evaluating the effect of interventions. They clearly can be applied to evaluation of some initiatives, but cannot be easily applied to all. For example, interventions that are not donor specific, such as advertising campaigns, are less amenable to RCT methodology. In addition, effort is required to plan recruitment activities so that they can be evaluated.

Pre-test/Post-test Design

When a RCT design is not possible, another alternative is a pre-test/post-test design. This is inherently weaker than a RCT because there is a chance that extraneous factors may have influenced the baseline measure (pre-test) and/or the after-intervention measure (post-test).

With a pre-test/post-test design, the number of donations is measured before an intervention and after the intervention. For example, the number of donations at a permanent collection site is known (the pre-test). Let's say a special intervention in the community is being implemented for a short period. It would be possible to count the number of units that were collected within a pre-determined time period and see if it was more than the baseline number. If the baseline measurement (the pre-test) is the same duration of time as the post-test immediately before the intervention, there is a chance that this measurement is lower or higher than normal, that is that it is not typical. However, if one counted the number units collected for several time periods of the same duration before the intervention was in place (and you may need to go back for a couple of years if there is seasonal variation), it will be possible to see if there is a discernable spike in units collected after the intervention. Because something else may have been happening in the community at the time (that perhaps recruiters are not aware of) this would be even better evaluated if the intervention were repeated after a while, and if a spike were again observed. Observing for a long enough period before and after the intervention, and repeating the intervention two or more times and observing the effect can mitigate some of the weakness of the design. However, if there are multiple initiatives underway at the same time, it still may not be possible to discern any independent effect.

Application for Strategy

It must be recognised that some very sound methodologies, such as the randomised controlled trial can be used in some circumstances but do not lend themselves to all initiatives that would be desirable to evaluate. However, randomised controlled trials are a good place to start when putting in place robust evaluative methods. The application of scientific methodology to evaluate the effectiveness of recruitment and retention interventions is a developing specialty. Creativity is needed to develop methods that are scientifically sound and operationally acceptable. Hence, in order to move towards an evidence-based recruitment and retention program, it must be recognised that how to evaluate will not always be obvious. Also, if the recruitment approach has been to implement a variety of activities with the key outcome being a target number of donations, that is to say, to be thankful that something that was done must have worked but not be overly concerned with teasing out *exactly* what worked, there is a substantial re-alignment of thinking necessary to make the commitment to coordinate activities to facilitate evaluation. Corporate strategy should focus on developing the expertise within the organization to be able to gather data in each of the three key areas – qualitative information, survey based methods and evaluation of recruitment/retention initiatives –but should pay special attention to developing knowledge amongst all recruitment staff, not just higher levels of management.

A process should be agreed upon which is based on the assessment phase and results in clear objective statements, and also describes what the information will be used for (which is essential for prioritising). This process should ensure that the focus stays on what is needed, not on what is easiest. In other words, don't let practical considerations limit thinking right from the 'get-go'. Once a decision has been made and it has been prioritised, then it is time to weigh up the practical considerations with the value of the information.

Strategies for Getting Evidence-Based Practice in Place

The preceding sections describe the types of information that can be drawn upon to facilitate evidence-based recruitment and retention initiatives, as well as some of the strengths and limitations of various forms of information or evidence. A blood establishment which has truly embraced evidence-based practice would have staff at all levels of the organization critically reading the literature, evaluating its generalizability to their own situation, conducting their own studies and analysis as appropriate and objectively evaluating what they do. One would expect that through this process, they would have some findings that would be of interest to the wider transfusion community and would be communicating their results in abstracts, presentations and most importantly in peer-reviewed publications.

Generally speaking, fresh new ideas have more potential to come from middle management and the front lines of recruitment staff than from senior management. This is because these are the people who are closest to the information and are able to focus on recruitment issues. Some top-down guidance is necessary, but the strategy should focus on building structures into the organization that will encourage creativity and foster evidence-based decision making among staff at all levels.

Staffing and Staff Development

Certainly every blood establishment needs personnel with expertise in research methods, in order to generate and organize information and evaluate practice. For a small organization, it may be most feasible to develop professional groups within the organization who share this function, but in large organizations a research unit may be appropriate.

Commitment to staff education, such as conference attendance or intensive courses in research design, will facilitate learning and creative thinking, and also communicate the commitment to evidence-based practice. This is important for senior staff, but extending such opportunities to others less senior is necessary to develop an evidence-based culture where it is most critical. Some seeding funds for small projects can stimulate creativity and a journal club - a regular meeting of staff that discusses the recent literature – is a good way to encourage critical thinking and enhance knowledge.

Staff Involvement in the Strategy Development

Perhaps the single most important determinant of success is the extent to which the strategic plan is seen as 'my plan' by the people who will implement it. Involving staff very early in the planning phase is essential, but it has to be real involvement. That is to say, staff input needs to be solicited and then it needs to be apparent that the plan was developed on this input. A sense of ownership over the strategic plan will only occur if staff can see real and tangible evidence that they developed the plan.

Assessment and Evaluation Are Part of the Job

There will be some degree of trial and error along the way and some staff performance indicators may decrease as skills are developing in evidence based practice. Evidence-based practice must become part of the performance upon which staff will be evaluated, and staff need to be able to see that efforts placed in this area are being recognized. If staff annual performance assessment is based primarily on such things as financial performance and unit collections, there is little incentive to 'go out on a limb' and try something new. Requiring staff to report the assessment and evaluation phases of their work is therefore extremely important. If evidence-based practice is to become an integral part of the recruitment and retention process, it needs to be recognized as work that has been done. In fact, if this is not done, it is unlikely that an evidence-based culture can be developed no matter how much effort is being placed in encouragement and resources.

Make Donor Data Accessible

Key data can be organized into internal web-based 'data cubes' which update as new data enters the database. 'Cubes' can be arranged according to topic. Using a 'point-and-click' approach, users can navigate the cubes with minimal training to bring up tables of data on their PC screen. With this arrangement up-to-date information on such things as collections by unit type, by blood type, by region, by donor demographics and by time frame (month and year) can be available to the entire organization.

Celebrate Success

Nothing succeeds like success! When someone demonstrates an evidence based approach to recruitment, it should be celebrated in some way within the organization. For example, a short article about the project could be circulated in the internal newsletter. The staff member could be asked to provide an in-service talk to other staff. It is helpful both as an example for others staff, and for demonstrating the high priority that evidence-based practice has in the organization.

Conclusion

Evidence-based donor recruitment and retention is a strategic approach to identifying 'how things are', and making decisions that support 'how things should be' and requires management to change the environment, not simply react to it. Evidence based practice means implementing a cyclic process of assessment, planning, implementation and evaluation in which the best scientific evidence available is used, and also collecting and evaluating data specific to the donors or general population of a blood center. Rigorous scientific evaluation of interventions is paramount to further assessment and planning.

There are essentially two aspects of strategy, therefore. Initially, a strategy to develop an organizational culture which embraces evidence-based practice, and is able to fully utilize evidence to develop recruitment strategy, must be planned and implemented. This will then enable strategic directions for recruitment and retention to be developed, based on thorough assessment of the evidence, and also to be modified. From the strategic directions specific interventions will arise. Based on scientific assessment that regularly examines the 'big picture', looking beyond short term gains, some groups of donors will be identified where much effort yields little gain, but for other groups a targeted approach may be more promising. This will challenge conventional beliefs and approaches about building and maintaining a viable donor base.

The ability of staff to evaluate published reports to identify strengths, limitations and application underpins evidence-based thinking. This essential skill set enables other evidence, much of which is available in most blood centers, to be optimally utilized. Evaluation of interventions is integral to an evidence-based approach – it will identify how effective the intervention was, and will provide direction in the next cycle of assessment. Methodology such as randomised controlled trials provides scientifically sound results, and although they cannot be applied in every situation, such methodology is an excellent place to start building an evidence-based approach. A key challenge is developing and/or refining evaluative methods that are practical and scientifically sound.

Strategy to develop evidence-based practice should focus principally on staff that actually do the recruiting and retaining of donors. Active and meaningful involvement of staff at all levels in the organization in strategic planning is extremely important, as is the availability of resources such as learning opportunities, easy access to donor data and access to research expertise. It should be noted that learning and applying scientific skills is a hurdle to be crossed initially, and especially until evaluative mechanisms become part of routine practice, extra effort is required by all. The best chances of success will be achieved if demonstrating evidence-based practice becomes 'part of the job' making it clear that effort in evidence-based approach will be recognised, and that success will be celebrated.

REFERENCES

[1] Piliavin JA, Callero PL. *Giving Blood: The Development of an Altruistic Identity.* Baltimore: John Hopkins University Press, 1991.
[2] Robinson EA, Murray A. Proceedings of the International Seminar, Royal College of Pathologists, 13 November 1998. Altruism: is it alive and well? *Transfus Med* 1999;9(4):351-82.
[3] Schreiber GB, Schlumpf KS, Glynn SA et al. Convenience, the bane of our existence, and other barriers to donating. *Transfusion* 2006;46(4):501-2.
[4] Sanchez AM, Ameti DI, Schreiber GB et al. The potential impact of incentives on future blood donation behavior. *Transfusion* 2001;41(2):172-8.
[5] Glynn SA, Schreiber GB, Murphy EL et al. Factors influencing the decision to donate: racial and ethnic comparisons. *Transfusion* 2006;46(6):980-90.
[6] Reich P, Roberts P, Laabs N et al. A randomized trial of blood donor recruitment strategies. *Transfusion* 2006;46(7):1090-6.
[7] Wu Y, Glynn SA, Schreiber GB. First-time blood donors: demographic trends. Transfusion 2001;41(3):360-4.
[8] Ownby HE, Kong F, Watanabe K et al. Analysis of donor return behaviour. Retrovirus Epidemiology Donor Study. *Transfusion* 1999;39(10):1128-35.
[9] Schreiber GB, Sharma UK, Wright DJ et al. First year donation patterns predict long-term commitment for first-time donors. *Vox Sang* 2005;88(2):114-21.
[10]Riley W, Schwei M, McCullogh J. The United States' potential blood donor pool: Estimating the prevalence of donor exclusion factors on the pool of potential donors *Transfusion* 2007;47(7):1180-88.
[11]Custer B, Johnson ES, Sullivan SD et al. Quantifying losses to the donated blood supply due to donor deferral and miscollection. *Transfusion* 2004;44(10):1417-26.
[12]Custer B, Chinn A, Hirschler NV, Busch MP, Murphy EL. The consequences of temporary deferral on future whole blood donation. *Transfusion* 2007;47(8):1514-23.
[13]Halperin D, Baetens J, Newman B. The effect of short-term, temporary deferral on future blood donation. *Transfusion* 1998;38(2):181-3.
[14]Chamla JH, Leland LS, Walsh K. Eliciting repeat blood donations: tell early career donors why their blood type is special and more will give again. Vox Sanguinis 2006;90(4):302-7.
[15]Zuck TF, Thomson RA, Schreiber GB et al. The Retrovirus Epidemiology Donor Study (REDS): rationale and methods. *Transfusion* 1995;35(11):944-51.

APPENDIX

Some Statistical and Data Collection Concepts

Some background in statistics and study design is pre-requisite to understanding this chapter. This section provides a very cursory look at some key concepts.

Inference

There are some occasions when the total number for a measurement of interest will be known, such as the total number of donors who made a donation over a particular time period. However, other than for very basic demographic data and donation dates, it is usually not practical to collect data on all donors. More frequently, one is able to collect data about a group of donors (a sample) but wishes to generalize this information to infer something about all donors. For example, if donor ethnic group data is not routinely collected, one might do a survey and use the data to estimate the proportion of different ethnic groups in the total donor base – that is make inference to the donor population from sample data. There are some special considerations for making inference from samples which should be considered prior to collecting the data as well as after the analysis

Ideal Sampling

The ideal donor sample should include:

1. Randomly selected donors such that every donor has an equal chance of being included in the sample. This is usually achieved by using a computer generated random list of the desired sample size drawn from a list of all donors.
2. Data should (ideally) be collected from every donor selected. Of course, not all donors will agree to participate, and it may not be possible to contact all donors on the list, but with more effort it is possible to get closer. For example, in a telephone survey it may take up to 10 attempts to contact the donor. Usually, it is possible to get at least 60% of donors to participate in a telephone survey, a little less for mail survey (with several mailings).
3. A large enough number of donors to ensure that donor responses or donor sub-groups can be accurately quantified.

Sampling Bias

Sampling bias occurs when the sample is not truly representative of the population from which it was derived, ant to which the findings are intended to be generalised. For example, if there were several mobile collection units in places where there were high concentrations of certain ethnic groups on the day of a survey at the collection sites, those groups will be over-represented and from the data it would be inferred that there are more donors from those ethnic groups than there really are. If the donors were selected randomly from a list, such as a computer generated list of all donors who made a donation over the past six months and then telephoned, then every donor has an equal chance of being selected and this reduces the sampling bias.

Response Bias

Response bias is another kind of bias and refers to donors self-selecting in some way to participate in the survey. For example, some donors from ethnic backgrounds may be less accustomed to completing questionnaires, and hence could be under-represented in the data that is collected, so that it will look like there are fewer donors from certain ethnic backgrounds than there really are. Response bias nearly always exists to some extent in survey data, but it can be minimised by 'working' the sample. For example, in a telephone survey, rather than leaving a message and hoping the donor will decide to call back, it is better to continue calling at different times and days until the donor can be asked in person. With this approach it will be possible to explain the importance of the survey, and encourage more donors to participate. For mail out surveys, some combination of mailing in series, such as an introductory letter first, and then mailing the questionnaire, and then mailing the questionnaire again if is not returned have been described and used for blood donor research to increase the response rate [15].

Sample Size

The sample needs to include enough donors to be confident that the sample accurately represents the donor population. Generally speaking, a larger sample will be more reflective of the donor population, but there will be a point where the sample is 'large enough' and the little extra precision that may be gained by including more donors is off-set by the cost and logistic difficulty of increasing the sample size further. Let's say that the true percentage of donors from a particular ethnic group is 1%. If data is collected from a very small number of donors, let's say 30, there is a much greater chance that this ethnic group will not be included in the sample at all, giving an estimate of 0%. If chance would have it that two such donors happened to be included in the sample then this would translate into 6.7%, and hence the proportion of donors from that ethnic group would be over-represented. The rarer something is, the larger the sample needs to be to provide an accurate estimate of the donor population. A statistician should be consulted to work out a suitable sample size.

Comparing Two (or more) Groups

If you randomly drew two samples of donors from the same pool of donors, likely they would have a somewhat different blend of ethnic groups, and the smaller the sample size of these two samples, the more likely differences are to be observed. In the above example it could be seen how one could easily have a point estimate of 0% or 6.7% in a sample of 30 donors drawn from the same donor population which had a true proportion of 1%.

When two groups of donors are compared, the real question is generally 'are these two groups of donors from different populations or the same population?' For example, if donors in two different cities were surveyed, do they have the same ethnic group distribution or different? The percentage of each ethnic group will be a little bit different, of course, because they are different samples and even if the two samples had been drawn from the same city they would be a little bit different. The two samples can be considered to be from different donor populations, (that the ethnic distribution is different between the two cities), if the probability that the variation observed in the two samples due to sampling is less than 5%, usually represented as $p<0.05$. This can be determined by a number of statistical tests.

In: Transfusion - Think About It
Editor: Trevor J. Cobain
ISBN 978-1-61668-969-8

Chapter 4

THE VALUE OF DATA IN THE DECISION MAKING PROCESS OF BLOOD PRODUCT PRODUCTION AND TRANSFUSION

Trevor J. Cobain and Alex Eigenstetter
South Eastern Area Laboratory Services (SEALS), South Eastern and Illawarra Area Health Service, Sydney, New South Wales, Australia.

ABSTRACT

The collection of accurate, current and readily adaptable data is essential for all areas of Transfusion Medicine.

For areas of production planning, maintenance of adequate stock, monitoring wastage or demonstrating appropriate or inappropriate usage and evaluating the effectiveness of products are all valid reasons for collecting data.

It may also be the case that the demand for this information has even more credence over the past decade as it has become more obvious that blood products are expensive even though many of them are donated. They are included in the budget of hospitals and are clearly a part of the cost for an episode in hospital and are also often in short supply.

Often the required data is not readily available. Computer systems may not have been designed with at least some of the requirements for collecting these data in mind.

The information described here considers some data that is useful both in the production end and the transfusion end of Transfusion Medicine. It gives two practical examples (one in Western Australia and one in New South Wales) when a system of linkage of critical patient identifiers was used to provide comprehensive information relating to how blood products were used.

This linkage method has been reproduced when PATHNET[3] was taken up by South Eastern Sydney and Illawarra Area Health Service (SESIAHS) during 2009 for the Blood Banks. By using unique identifiers including: medical record number, date of birth, Surname, Given Name and dates and time it is possible to link transfusion information

[3] Cerner Corporation, 2800 Rockcreek Parkway, Kansas City, MO 64117, USA.

including type and number of product to other laboratory systems, doctor requesting, ward and also to clinical information including ICD-10 codes.

None of the computers or the software were specifically designed for collecting such data and the computer systems were quite different between the two States.

This is a valuable model for a method of how to collect data that is essential to better understand and monitor how blood products are produced and used.

INTRODUCTION

The availability of accurate and comprehensive data is essential within the various sections of Transfusion Medicine [1-11]. When the information technology systems are adaptable or have been specifically designed for these purposes the data may be readily available. Much of the data has been directed at making sure that there are no inappropriate transfusions and that every blood product that is transfused is "safe". There is always an expectation from the donor that the donation will be fully utilized and from the recipient that the blood product is totally safe. In spite of the many challenges that have been evident in Transfusion Medicine (particularly over the past 15 years) and the serious immunological and non-immunological complications red cell transfusion holds, a therapeutic index that exceeds many of the common medications has been achieved [12]. However, many of the systems that are currently available may not have this versatility. The aim of this chapter is to clearly identify some of the data that is useful and to give examples of how useful information may be obtained even if the computing software has not been specifically written for this purpose.

For simplicity the data will be considered as two sections:

Those that are particularly relevant to the Blood Service that is producing the products.

And:

Data that will enable some evaluation of the way Blood Products are being transfused. Data directly related to the Hospital Transfusion Unit.

THE BLOOD SERVICE

These data may be useful in their own right but may also be required to be considered in conjunction with other information. In particular they may be considered with information such as financial costing, staffing levels, population statistics, and hospital activities etc [13-15].

Donor Demographics information is essential. This has been documented extensively previously [16-20] and is the subject of an additional chapter in this book by Sheila O'Brien. It is suffice therefore to indicate that in these situations data relating to distribution of donors in a population, the number of donations per year, the aged distribution of donors, the factors influencing donor response and behaviours and the response of changes in regulatory requirements are all issues that require reliable and up-to-date data if the Blood Service is to respond adequately to demand for blood products.

How the donation is used is very important from many aspects. It is very important to ensure that the donation is used efficiently for the reasons of an adequate stock inventory but there is also a very strong expectation by the donor that their valuable donation has not been wasted in any way.

All through the donation process there is a continual decision relating to whether or not the donor and the donation can be fully utilised, partially utilised or not used at all.

It is also useful to have information relating to what type of donation has been collected from the donor as this may have implications on the production schedule and the number of donors required. Examples relating to this are given by the comparison of aphaeresis collections versus whole blood collections. It is evident that one aphaeresis collection of platelets may be equivalent to four or five platelets collected from whole blood, similarly the volume of plasma collected by aphaeresis maybe approximately 600ml whereas the volume of plasma collected from a whole blood donation may only be 250 or 290ml. These types of differences can make major differences in the number of donors required to maintain adequate supplies of blood products-particularly in the case of platelet production when the lifespan of the product is only five days and there may be a requirement to rapidly boost production. It is also essential that adequate investigation and data becomes available to identify the blood products of choice. Even though platelet products contain similar number of platelets it is important to understand if these are comparable in their outcome [21-23]. Similarly it is important to understand if there is a requirement for blood products such as "warm whole blood" – even if the logistics and costs may be more during the production phase [24,25]. This is very difficult to decide if the data is not available for valid comparison. Both of these are very important issues during the planning of Blood Transfusion Medicine and constitute a specific chapter in this book.

Table 1 given below can best demonstrate these data:

From Table 1 it is clear that the process is rather complicated and it's not a matter of having the choice of producing whatever is required from any donation. Some donations can only be used to make limited products. This is usually related to safety or regulatory issues. Quite a large proportion of donors may be rejected or deferred for similar reasons. In addition some products may be discarded during some stage of production. This may be because additional information has become available (such as laboratory testing) or there may have been some issue during production that limits the products use.

All of these data are required to monitor and to improve efficiency of production. In addition, there are major differences between the data for whole blood and aphaeresis collections. It is also evident that the aphaeresis collection varies during the nine months that have been selected during 2001/2002. This is mainly because aphaeresis collections are relatively costly and are planned and collected for specific products and often are used to boost production for particular products. In addition it is clear that the rate of rejection or the wastage is proportionately less for aphaeresis compared to whole blood donors. This is at least in part due to the fact that the aphaeresis donors returned more regularly than whole blood donors and are to some extent more selected than whole blood donors. The aphaeresis donors are more likely to have veins that are more readily entered for blood donation. In addition the aphaeresis donation is more likely to be decided upon what is required rather than what can be produced from a basic, whole blood donation.

The next important stage of the production and use of Blood Products is the period of storage prior to a decision to use the products or not. This stage may occur at either the Blood Service or the Transfusion Unit. Table 2 summarizes the outcome of the products in these situations. The availability of these data are heavily reliant on the relationship of the Blood service and the Transfusion Unit. It is also essential that there is frequent, open and constructive discussion relating to these data between these organisations if efficiency is to be maintained.

Table 1.

Blood Use code data for 2001-02 Blood Use Code	Jul-01	Aug-01	Sep-01	Oct-01	Nov-01	Dec-01	Jan-02	Feb-02	Mar-02	Total
Full Use	4577	4390	4223	4582	4571	4373	4807	4324	3967	39814
Red cells + Plasma	772	778	704	762	711	724	752	674	596	6473
Red cells only	9	1	0	0	0	0	0	0	0	10
Plasma only	782	840	754	812	823	747	805	743	668	6974
Deferred/rejected	799	745	791	742	721	681	726	619	574	6398
Test only	155	177	154	162	184	166	200	196	189	1583
No bag no test	65	74	81	75	75	69	83	90	79	691
Donation but no test	83	82	74	73	70	85	92	73	63	695
Discard all (prior to processing)	263	290	315	323	272	331	261	212	219	2486
Discard all (after processing)	13	21	25	44	36	23	35	35	23	255
Total unusable product	1378	1389	1440	1419	1358	1355	1397	1225	1147	12108
Auto/Directed	131	116	107	127	145	69	138	131	118	1082
Plasmapheresis	1250	1334	1151	1365	1597	1337	1511	1564	1615	12724
Aphaeresis plts + plasma	374	383	355	377	404	361	347	354	347	3302
Aphaeresis plts only	4	10	1	4	9	4	6	5	10	53
Total Aphaeresis (Usable)	1628	1727	1507	1746	2010	1702	1864	1923	1972	16079
Aphaeresis deferred/rejected										
Test only	4	3	4	8	9	6	7	4	10	55
No bag no test	0	0	1	0	0	0	0	1	1	3
Donation but no test										
Discard all (prior to processing)	11	4	3	8	6	12	6	9	7	66
Discard all (after processing)	9	5	4	20	5	8	5	9	9	74
Total unusable product	24	12	12	36	20	26	18	23	27	198
Total	9301	9253	8747	9484	9638	8996	9781	9043	8495	82738

The data included here is an accumulation of outcomes from both the Blood Service and the Transfusion Unit. For instance, expiry may have occurred at either location although the majority of expiry was in the hospitals. The "Unaccounted" outcome was exclusively in the hospitals as the Blood Service relied on the Hospitals to identify what was the final outcome of each blood product. If this was unknown a month after expiry, the hospital was specifically asked for an outcome. If this was not forthcoming the product was listed as Unaccounted.

Table 2.

July 02 –June 03					
	Transfused	**Expired**	**Discarded**	**Out of Fridge**	**Unaccounted**
Autologous Red\Cells	757	121	16	5	15
Autologous WB	63	1	1	0	2
Total Autologous Red Cells	820	122	17	5	17
Homologous Red Cells	31821	3993	713	143	598
Homologous WB	334	15	11	10	0
Frozen/Washed/Filtered Red Cells	19811	229	168	5	104
Paediatric Red Cells	512	833	992	4	31
Total Homologous Red Cells	52478	5070	1884	162	733
WB Platelets	2096	911	25	0	22
Aph Platelets	5522	589	32	0	94
Total Platelets	7618	1500	57	0	116
Clinical Plasma	11276	156	601	0	142
Cryoprecipitate	1741	137	124	0	34

It should be emphasised that there are many variables that have some effect on these data. The products included in Table 2 included those from all over Western Australia. The Regional areas of this part of Australia are small and very remote. Transport into these areas is limited and therefore the stocks of products are such that they need to cover many contingencies in the knowledge that additional supplies may not be available for at least 24 hours. The characteristics of the various products have also had some visible affects on these data. The mix of blood groups is not included in Table 2 but is obviously a contributor to how blood products are utilized. The life span of the products is very important. A comparison between platelets (5 day expiry) and fresh frozen plasma (1 year) is to have an impact on "waste". The products that are included in this table are varied and it could be argued that they are used to varying degrees of efficiency. 97.5% of filtered or washed red cells are transfused compared with 85.3% of the standard red cells and only 21.6% of paediatric red cells. Some of this difference may be reflecting education of the staff who are using these products in that they understand that filtered red cells are expensive to produce and therefore need to be used very efficiently or they maybe used as they are seen to be better products and are therefore used in preference. In any event, at this time, the filtered product was still less in number to the unfiltered products. To some extent a similar argument may be directed towards aphaeresis platelets compared with the whole blood derived platelets.

The situation relating to the Paediatric Red Cells was complex. At the time 5 small volume red cell units were produced from one red cell donation for paediatric use. Policy at that time required that the paediatric products from one donor would only be transfused to one recipient. This meant that if only one unit was required the other 4 would be discarded. The data from Table 2 was very useful in evaluating product use and was instrumental in a revision of the way in which paediatric red cells were produced so that it greatly improved the efficiency.

INFORMATION AT THE HOSPITAL TRANSFUSION UNIT

The data available from the Transfusion Unit can be used for multiple purposes. It may be rather basic with an efficiency bias. Data in this category may include stock levels or some of the data that has been included above.

Table 3 indicates some examples of the data relating to the stock level.

Table 3.

	HOSPITAL STOCK HOLDINGS															
Hospital/ Location (Coded)	Red Blood Cells								Clinical FFP				Cryo			
	O Pos	O Neg	A Pos	A Neg	B Pos	B Neg	AB Pos	AB Neg	O	A	B	AB	O	A	B	AB
A	50	12	50	15	15	6	6	6	24	24	24	24	2	2	1	1
B	25	12	25	10	10	4	8	4	10	10	10	6	3	3	3	
C	20	10	20	7	6	3	4	2	8	8	8	8	2	2	1	1
D	6	6	6	2	2	1	1	1				4				1
E	40	12	40	15	10	6	6	6	14	14	14	14	4	4	4	2
F	10	6	6													
G	6	4	4													
H	10	6	10	6	6				4	4	4	4	1	1	1	
I	17	12	15	4	2		4		4	4	4	4	1	1	1	
J	20	6	20	10	5	3	2		6	6	4	4	1	1		
K	20	6	20	10	4	2	2		6	6	4	4	1	1		
L	20	10	15	8	8	2	4		4	4	4	2	1	1	1	
M	16	8	10	4	0	0	0	0	0	0		12				1
O	20	10	20	6					2	2		10				1
P	20	10	20	6					8	8	4	10				1
Q	6	4	4	0	0	0	0	0	0	0	0	0	0	0	0	0
R	6	4	4	0	0	0	0	0	0	0	0	4	0	0	0	0

The extent of the stock holding may be an agreement between the Blood Service and the Transfusion Unit. It will be a required mixture of blood products and an agreed mix of groups. This suggests that there is some understanding of the population that the Hospital is servicing and some understanding of what is reasonable for the Blood Service to provide given that some blood groups are more difficult to locate and some acceptance that there may be a requirement to utilize blood that is compatible but not necessarily of identical group – particularly for some products from time to time. There may also be some special considerations to take into account based on the distance the Hospital/ Transfusion Unit is from a reliable supply of additional blood products. It should also be recognised that some of these issues have been made more complex or demanding with some of the more stringent requirements for blood product storage and transportation that may have had a definite affect on the protocols involved in the Issue, Return of blood to the Blood Service and the Re-issue of blood products as well as the exchange of blood products between Hospitals or Transfusion Units without the direct involvement of the Blood Service.

The way in which an agreed stock level is used may vary. In an ideal situation there may be some "real time" data that is available to the Blood service – that is some electronic means of determining how closely the current blood stocks at a Hospital compares to an agreed stock level. However, this is a fairly rare situation and requires a particular relationship between the Hospital and the Blood Service. In many situations the way in which this data is obtained may be by some form of specific communication between these organizations at predetermined intervals. The agreed level of stock holding may be affected by the distance from the available blood stocks and may also be influenced by the number of stock deliveries for any period of time. Maybe not surprisingly these two factors also have some impact on how efficiently the stocks of blood are used. The mix of group is important to how efficiently blood is used. There maybe valid reasons why some remote hospitals should have a stock of O negative blood. The question may well be asked if it may be more efficient to provide a larger number of O negative rather that a mix of B pos, neg, A pos neg etc. This question may also be related to whether it is reasonable to consider directing a large proportion of AB donors into aphaeresis plasma production rather than into whole blood and red cell production when the AB red cells frequently expire in the hospitals.

Additional Information from the Transfusion Unit may be more complex. This can be in several forms:

Comprehensive Epidemiological or Demographical Data

The Demographic information is very useful for planning and to some extent being able to compare various populations.

Sex and age distribution of the recipient population may be important information when planning for the future or predicting the production level for blood products. The number of products transfused per hospital stay or transfusion episode may provide useful data when expressed as a distribution frequency. The number of products transfused per patient and the total number of patients who are recipients of the transfusion of the blood products may be a marker to efficiency and may be a rather crude but useful way of making comparison between populations. The number of products transfused/ 100,000 population is also a marker that gives some comparison between populations. When the sample is large it may be useful for comparison and is useful when comparing the use of various blood products between countries [26]. This may also be a useful marker but needs to be taken in the context of the available resources of the countries being compared. These are sometimes very difficult data to obtain. Many organisations may not have the facilities to collect blood use data for a total population or a "captive" population which is required if calculating use per 100,000 population. In many situations patients may be referred from places distant to the location in which the service is provided. This may then mean that comparisons between such facilities need to be compared with caution and the definition of the population needs to be complete.

Data which Relates to Guidelines

There have been many techniques that have been employed to modify or influence blood product use [27-43]. One such method has been to introduce guidelines [44-56]. In Australia the guidelines come from the NHMRC/ASBT [57]. There are many others. Most will outline Laboratory parameters (usually with some rider for a particular clinical situation) at which point transfusion is indicated. For instance the ANZSBT Guidelines suggest a cut off of

120g/L of Haemoglobin for a red cell transfusion and a platelet count of 50 x 10^9/L for a platelet transfusion. The guidelines for plasma and cryoprecipitate are probably less defined but may relate to the International Normalized Ratio (INR) for plasma and fibrinogen concentration for cryoprecipitate.

Having established these guidelines it can be relatively complicated to determine if they are being followed or what the level of compliance is. It may be that the laboratory parameters are expected on the form requesting the blood product. This may be ideal but is very difficult to achieve – particularly in situations of "urgent" transfusion. Some have endeavoured to collect data retrospectively by examining patient headsheets. This is very time consuming and most of the studies relating to these types of data are understandably of fairly small numbers.

An alternative method of obtaining this information is discussed later in this chapter.

More Detailed Information Relating to the Transfusion Event

There is a very wide range of other clinical information, relating to the patient and the episode in hospital, that has triggered the transfusion.

The location within a specific hospital, a specific ward or location within a hospital. This is important from the point of view of planning production but also may be useful if at some stage it becomes possible to compare similar procedures or diseases between wards or hospitals. It may seem surprising that this data is not always available because the products must have been issued somewhere, however the data may not always be retrievable.

Being able to locate and analyse the details of products transfused is also very important for the same reasons as above. It is very important to have these data available particularly when evaluating any differences that may be seen in the location of blood product transfusion. Such situations arise when analysing data for patients who are of different sizes (such as children, babies, different racial groups) and also where product that are transfused are of different volume or quality (such as aphaeresis Vs whole blood platelets, varying volume of clinical plasma and red cells or whole blood).

It is reasonable to expect that all of the data for the examples listed below could be available so that reasonable and justifiable decisions can be made:

Demographics

The age and sex mix of the patients receiving particular products.

The distribution of number of products transfused/ episode.

The number of products produced, issued, transfused.

How many patients are involved for a number of products transfused?

Following Guidelines?

What proportion of patients has the expected Laboratory tests?
What is the Haemoglobin concentration immediately before Red Cell transfusion?
Platelet Count immediately prior to and after Platelet transfusion.
INR to monitor Plasma transfusion
Fibrinogen to monitor Cryoprecipitate transfusion

More Detailed Information Relating to the Transfusion Event

Location within a specific hospital, specific ward/ location within a Hospital
Details of products transfused
Specific medical staff/Specialty
Specific for a patient
Specific for an episode in Hospital
Procedure involved
Disease involved

Extra Information may be Useful and Desirable

Length of stay
Time in ICU
Returned to theatre?
Other procedures that may affect blood product use such as particular drug use or procedures such as salvage.
Indication of outcome eg death or otherwise

Some Measure of National Comparison

May be useful to compare/benchmark with other countries
The number of products transfused/100,000 population
Compare distribution of products based on Diagnostic Related Groups (or similar)

There are particular challenges relating to the collection of much of these data. Obviously there is a genuine requirement to protect the privacy of the patients and the donors. This is something that must be considered frequently and often the exclusion of name from the analysed data may not be sufficient particularly if a patient is undergoing an unusual procedure on a particular date in a relatively small city.

There also appears to be an expectation from some of the other institutions involved in the production and use of blood products that these type of data are "Commercial and in Confidence" or have the potential to adversely affect their operation if the data is freely available. Many of these institutions are providing a service for the population and are often funded by the public coffers. In Australia, the cost of some blood products has only recently become available. It is very difficult to produce a true total cost of a procedure if the cost of all blood products is limited and if the costs are set by the institution that produces the products in a monopoly situation.

For all of the reasons outlined above the data in this book has been carefully considered and presented in such a way to minimise jeopardising any of these sensitivities.

There are some Transfusion Centres and Blood Services that may have information technology systems that allow the collection of most of these data. However, this may not always be the case.

To determine the required information it has often required extremely time consuming searches through patient head sheets or other records. In some situation this has either meant that it was a situation that could only occur as a "once off" or very rarely or alternatively it included only a sample of transfusions – often of fairly small numbers.

Below are two examples that include procedures to use linkage of transfusion data to other laboratory or Hospital data in such a way that it has the utility to answer many of the questions posed above. This is a process that may well be available in many Blood Services and Hospitals elsewhere.

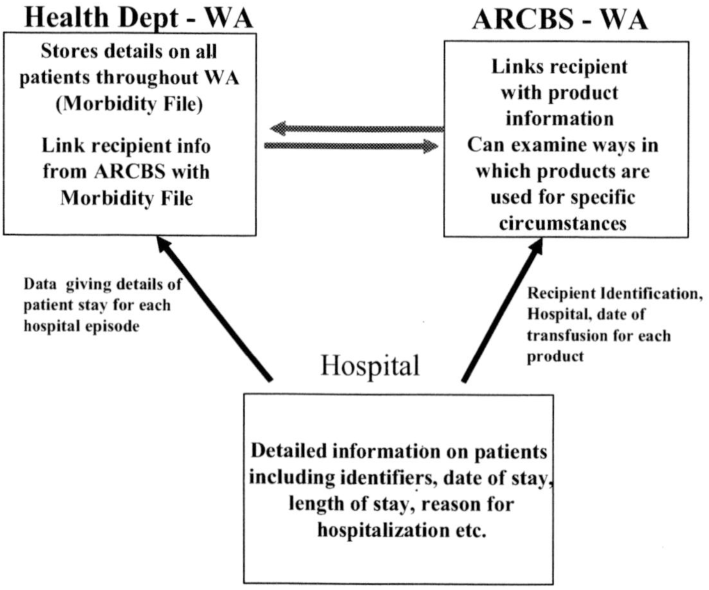

Figure 1. represents data that was collected in Western Australia. The process was as outlined. Data for transfusions throughout Western Australia was returned to the Blood Service. This included the date of transfusion, the identification of the patient and the product transfused. This information was then linked to the Morbidity Files that were available in the Health Department of Western Australia. If they were able to be linked to a particular hospital episode (within three days of the transfusion date) it was assumed that the transfusion was related with the particular disease or procedure associated with that hospital visit.

Some of the data has been published previously [58]. The procedure was such that it was able to produce data for a complete year and data for the entire Western Australian population, including the Regional hospitals in remote Western Australia. The procedure was sufficiently reproducible that it enabled the procedure to be duplicated for several years. The comparison for these years is also given below (Table 4).

Table 4. Summary of Available Data from Western Australia

	YEAR			
	1994/95	1996/97	2000/01	2001/02
Total Products Transfused	72041	80709	67448	71256
Products Linked	62169	74286	66904	69814
% Linked	86.3	92.0	99.2	98.0

The procedure was similar during the four years for which data was collected. The linkage process was refined during this period and it can be seen that it improved from 86.3% in 1994/95 to close to 100% during 2000/2002.

One of the limitations of the procedure was when the hospitals refused to supply the information relating to transfusion. Because the Blood Service provided all of the products for transfusion it was possible to monitor this outcome. During 2001/02, after following up unaccounted for products, the products that were issued but were unavailable for linkage was approximately 2% (Table 5). This was in addition to the number of products that could not be linked to the Morbidity Files.

Table 5. Details of Linkage (2001/02 (WA))

Information returned by all hospitals
Unaccounted products investigated further
During 2000/01, Approx. 2% unaccounted
During 2000/01 71256 products transfused
69814 linked to Morbidity files

The data relating to this linkage process has been published elsewhere and is not presented here other than to summarise the number of blood products, the number of transfusion episodes (transfusion during one hospital visit) and the number of patients involved in transfusion for the whole of Western Australia during the financial year 2001/02 (Table 6).

Table 6. Number Products, Episodes and Patients (2001/02 (WA))

	Total Products	*Number Episodes*	*Number Patients*
Red Cells	50605	16674	11016
WB Platelets	2734	473	448
Aph Platelets	5050	2170	1276
Total Platelets	7784	2407	1475
Plasma	9642	2207	1980
Total	69814	18070*	11692*

* Totals may not add up. Several products are represented in the same Episode.

The other example of data that is obtained from utilizing linkage is obtained from data collected in New South Wales. The data was collected from information technology systems that were completely unrelated and running different software.

The data originated from a major transfusion centre that serviced several hospitals on one site in a Sydney suburb. The data originally identified the patient and the blood product transfused. It was possible to then match and link this with the haematology laboratory parameters (such as Haemoglobin, Platelets Count and INR) for a similar Medical Record Number for the day before or the day of the transfusion. Some records had more than one laboratory result for a particular day. In these circumstances the first result was included in the analysis. It was also then possible to link the transfusion information to the Medical Records system so that clinical and other information relating to the transfusion and the hospital stay could be associated. This was possible for all transfusions that were performed on this site for the complete year of 2005/06.

This procedure produced data that listed the use of all blood products for the hospital site and included the use by the four hospitals on the site and enabled the use to identify all of the wards involved. Data was collected for all of the processed products (Albumex, Intragam etc) as well as the fresh blood products but only data relating to Red cells, Platelets and Plasma is included here.

Table 7. Product Summary 2005/06

	Number Issued	*Number Transfused*	*Number of Patients*
Total	23947	22480	2972*
Red Cells	15867	15331	2760
Plasma	3350	3010	672
Platelets	2982	2468	601
Cryoprecipitate	1573	1508	131
Cryosupernatant	175	163	3

* Many patients transfused with more than one product.

A summary of the total data is given in Table 7. A total of 22480 transfusions were performed during 2005/06. Not all of the blood products issued were transfused. One of the limitations of the current process is indicated by the number of patients. It was clear that a significant number of the patients involved in transfusion returned several times during the year for multiple transfusion events.

Table 8. Summary of Transfused Red Cells

15331 Transfused
4688 had no Hb result
10603 Hb 1 day before or day of transfusion
40 no Hb but other Haematology
2794 Hb > 100g/L (26%)

The summary of the Red Cell transfusions indicate that the Guidelines of the NHMRC/ASBT may not have been met in a large proportion (Table 8). 4688 transfusions were performed without a Haemoglobin measurement and 2794 were above the recommended concentration of 100g/L at the time of transfusion.

There was also some difference between the way in which various wards used Haemoglobin measurement to determine the justification of red cell transfusion (Table 9). This is still being investigated but it is reasonable to acknowledge that the difference is marked in some instances. The data marked with an asterisk (*) highlights outliers in Tables 9 and 11.

Table 9. Location Transfusing Red Cells with Hb > 100g/L 2005/06

	Number	*Total Trans*	*% of Trans*
Ward 1	494	2074	23.8
Ward 2	320	660	48.5*
Ward 3	187	714	26.1
Ward 4	154	508	30.3
Ward 5	115	916	12.6
Ward 6	101	1155	8.7
Ward 7	99	418	23.7
Ward 8	95	261	36.4
Ward 9	89	587	15.2

Similarly with platelet transfusion (Table 10), there were some occasions when a transfusion was performed without a platelet count although the percentage was much higher (94.6%) compared with the red cell transfusions (69.1%). Although this may also be reflecting the fact that the red cell transfusions often included many units transfused where as the platelets were most often a single dose.

There was also considerable variability between the wards of when a platelet transfusion was performed (Table 11). One ward implemented transfusion in >90% of their patients with a platelet count of >50 x 10^9/L where as another ward transfused in only 10% of patient with a platelet count of >50 x 10^9/L.

Table 10. Summary of Transfused Platelets

2468 Transfused
129 had no Platelet Count
2336 Platelet Count 1 day before or day of transfusion
3 no Platelet Count but other Haematology
726 Platelet Count > 50 x 10^9/L (31%)

There was little laboratory evidence for plasma transfusion in that approximately 30% had no testing prior to the transfusion and almost 50% of those tested had laboratory parameters that were outside the NHMRC/ASBT guidelines (Table 12).

Table 11. Location Transfusing Platelets with Count > 50 x 10^9/L 2005/2006

	Number	*Total Transfusions*	*% of Transfusions*
Ward 1	153	163	93.9*
Ward 2	88	97	90.7
Ward 3	82	770	10.6*
Ward 4	67	230	29.1
Ward 5	48	93	51.6
Ward 6	22	27	81.5
Ward 7	21	37	56.8
Ward 8	21	33	63.6
Ward 9	17	39	43.6

Table 12. Summary of Transfused Plasma

3010 Transfused
1013 no laboratory testing
1986 had an INR 1 day before or day of transfusion
1997 had an APTT 1 day before or day of transfusion
921 < 1.5 INR (46%)

After analysing these data it was also considered that it would be useful to continue the linkage system to combine these data with some clinical information that was available on the morbidity files that were available for the South Eastern Sydney and Illawarra Area Health Service (SESIAHS). To this end a pilot study was performed on the 2005/06 data from a hospital for women that was located in this area. Data was collected from the second 6 months of the 2005/06 year.

The data were linked if the blood product issue date matched between the episode start and end dates relating to the morbidity data. The linked file included Principle and subsequent diagnosis codes, MDC, DRG and Principle Procedure and subsequent procedure codes. Many of the other data included in the Morbidity files were also included.

Of the 440 records that were available for linkage only one did not match and was excluded from the linkage procedure. All of the data as described above was still available and comprehensive information relating to outcome, length of stay and specific clinical information was also available. A summary of the available data is given in Table 13. As indicated above there were a total of 439 red cells that were transfused in this example of the data. This represented 167 episodes in hospital and 155 different patients. It is therefore evident that some of the patients attended for more than one episode during this trial of the data linkage. Table 13 also indicates the number of units of red cells that were transfused during each episode and also how many units of red cells were transfused to each of the patients during this period.

Table 13. Summary of Data Linked to the Morbidity Files 2005/2006

Number of Red Cells Transfused	*Number of Patients*	*Number of Episodes*
1	36	41
2	54	63
3	25	28
4	22	19
5	6	5
6	2	2
7	2	3
8	1	2
9	4	3
10	1	0
11	2	1
Total	155	167

Some additional data that can be obtained by these methods are given below:

Table 14 lists the major Diagnosis Related Groups for the women who received Red Cell Transfused at this hospital during the second half of 2005/06. Table 15 also lists the Neonates who were transfused during a similar period. Much of the coded information for the neonates was limited and additional investigation is required to improve this set of data.

Table 16 indicates information relating to patient outcome. This is very useful when comparing or when deciding which blood product is optimal for a preferred patient outcome.

Table 17 indicates the Haemoglobin for the patients in this hospital during 2005/06 and who received a transfusion of red cells. They have been divided into the female, adult patients and the patient who were born at the hospital. It is very clear that the Haemoglobin distribution of the two groups is quite different. The adult women have a much larger proportion in the range for less than 70 to 90 g/L. It is clear that a much larger proportion of the paediatric patients would be outside the NHMRC/ASBT Guidelines for Red Cell transfusion. However, an alternative interpretation is that these guidelines may not completely satisfy the paediatric population.

Table 14.

DRG Description	
20 to 89 Years	
DRG Description	Number
Obstetrics Related	130
Malignancy	91
Gynaecology	66
Gastroenterology	16
Other	16
Total	319

Table 15.

DRG Description	
Less than or Equal to 1 Year old	
Birth Weight (g)	Number
<750	32
750 to 999	43
1000 to 1499	14
1500 to 1999	13
2000 to 2499	3
>2499	12
Other	3
Total	120

Table 16.

Patients receiving Red Cell Transfusion During 2005/06		
	Women Age (20 to 89 Years)	Babies (less or equal 1 Year)
Mode of Separation	Number	Number
Discharged by Hospital	287	65
Transferred to another hospital	25	49
Death without autopsy	5	6
Transferred to Palliative Care	2	0
Total	319	120

Table 17.

Patients receiving Red Cell Transfusion During 2005/06		
	Women Age (20 to 89 Years)	Babies (less or equal 1 Year)
Haemoglobin at Transfusion (g/L)	Percent of Those Transfused	Percent of Those Transfused
Less or Equal 70	14.1	1.7
>70 to 80	18.5	9.9
>80 to 90	22.1	15.2
>90 to 100	15	31.8
>100 to 110	9.1	13.3
>110 to 120	12.3	6.6
>120 to 130	4.1	9.9
>130 to 140	2.4	4.1
>140 to 150	1.5	1.7
>150 to 160	0.9	3.3
>160 to 170	0	1.7
>170 to 180	0	0
>180 to 190	0	0.8
Total	100	100

Conclusion

It is becoming more important that suitable and reliable data is available for many aspects of Transfusion Medicine. With more stringent requirements placed on donor selection and an expectation that blood products are used sparingly there is a requirement that those who use blood products can demonstrate justification for their use and to be able to compare one clinician transfusing blood products with another. Until recently, in some countries (including Australia) blood products were often thought of as "free". This is no longer the situation. The cost of blood products has become a significant issue throughout health systems and is widely acknowledged as being a major contributing factor to the overall cost of a patient's hospital stay.

There is also a wide range of reasons why data is essential for running a Transfusion system from the planning of the donation to the final outcome for the patient and even at the time of "lookback" during adverse consequences.

The fact is that not all of the Blood Services and the Transfusion units have Information Technology systems that are user friendly to the point where they can provide all of the information that is required and is in a situation that it can adapt for the ever changing requirements of modern transfusion medicine. What we have proposed here may not be the ideal situation but it is a system that has considerable utility and can be adapted to many of the requirements that are likely to be demanded. It is based on some requirements that are often readily available within basic systems. The unique identifier of the patient and the date of transfusion are two of the major requirements for the linkage systems that have been highlighted here as being successfully implemented in both Western Australia and in New South Wales with totally different sets of data and using variable computer resources. It is proposed that these are essential tools in striving to obtain the optimal blood product and to use it as efficiently as the donor would expect and as safely as the patient will demand.

References

[1] Rubin GL, Schofield WN, Dean MG, Shakeshaft AP. Appropriateness of red cell transfusion in major urban hospitals and effectiveness of an intervention. *Med J Aust.* 2001 175(7): 354-358.

[2] Schofield WN, Rubin GL, Dean MG. Appropriateness of platelet, fresh frozen plasma and cryoprecipitate transfusion in New South Wales public hospitals. *Med J Aust.* 2003 178(3): 117-121.

[3] Glynn A, McCarthy T, McCarroll M, Murray P. A prospective audit of blood usage post primary total knee arthroplasty. *Acta Orthop Belg.* 2006 72(1): 24-28.

[4] Grey DE, Smith V, Villanueva G, Richards B, Augustson B, Erber WN. The utility of an automated electronic system to monitor audit transfusion practice. *Vox Sang.* 2006 90(4): 316-324.

[5] Friedman MT, Ebrahim A. Adequacy of physician documentation of red blood cell transfusion and correlation with assessment of transfusion appropriateness. *Arch Pathol Lab Med.* 2006 130(4): 474-479.

[6] Sorensen BS, Johnsen SP, Jorgensen J. Complications related to blood donation: a population study. *Vox Sang*. 2007 Nov 19 [Epub ahead of print]

[7] Reilly M, Szulkin R. Statistical analysis of donation-transfusion data with complex correlation. *Stat Med*. 2007 26(30): 5572-5585.

[8] Katsaliaki K. Cost-effective practice in the blood service sector. *Health Policy* 2007 Dec. 24 [Epub ahead of print].

[9] Turgeon AF, Fergusson Da, Doucette S, Khanna MP, Tinmouth A, Aziz A, Hebert PC. Red blood cell transfusion practice amongst Canadian anesthesiologists: a survey. *Can J Anaesth*. 2006 53(4): 344-352.

[10] Greinacher A, Fendrich K, Alpen U, Hoffmann W. Impact of demographic changes on the blood supply: Mecklenburg-West Pomerania as a model region for Europe. *Transfusion* 2007 47(3): 395-401.

[11] Brace V, Kernaghan D, Penney G. Learning from adverse clinical outcomes: major obstetric haemorrhage in Scotland, 2003-05. *BJOG* 2007 114(11): 1388-1396.

[12] Klein HG, Spahn DR, Carson JL. Red blood cell transfusion in clinical practice. *Lancet* 2007 370(9585):415-426.

[13] Blanchette CM, Wang PF, Joshi AV, Kruse P, Asmussen M, Saunders W. Resource utilization and cost of blood management services associated with knee and hip surgeries in US hospitals. *Adv Ther*. 2006 23(1): 54-67.

[14] Blanchette CM, Joshi AV, Szpalski M, Gunzburg R, Du Bois M, Donceel P, Saunders WB. Comparison between spinal surgery blood transfusion service costs and associated treatment practices in the United States and Belgium. *Curr Med Opin*. 2007 23(11):2793-2804.

[15] Martinez V, Monsaingeon-Leon A, Cherif K, Judet T, Chauvin M, Fletcher D. Transfusion strategy for primary knee and hip arthroplasty : impact of an algorithm to lower transfusion rátes and hospital cost. *Br J Anaesth*. 2007 99(6): 794-800.

[16] Godin G, Conner M, Sheeran P, Belanger-Gravel A, Germain M. Determinants of repeated blood donation among new and experienced blood donors. *Transfusion* 2007 47(9): 1607-1615.

[17] France JL, France CR, Himawan LK. A path analysis of intention to redonate among experience blood donors: an extension of the theory of planned behaviour. *Transfusion* 2007 47(6): 1006-1013.

[18] Schlumpf KS, Glynn SA, Schreiber GB, Wright DJ, Randolph Steele W, Tu Y, Hermansen S, Higgins MJ, Garratty G, Murphy EL, National Heart Lung and Blood Institute Retrovirus Epidemiology Donor Study. Factors influencing donor return. *Transfusion* 2007 Nov 13 [Epub ahead of print].

[19] Steele WR, Schreiber GB, Guiltinan A, Nass C, Glynn SA, Wright DJ, Kessler D, Schlumpf KS, Tu Y, Smith JW, Garratty G, Retrovirus Epidemiolgy Donor Study. *Transfusion* 2007 Sep 25 [Epub ahead of print].

[20] Zou S, Musavi F, Notari EP 4th, Fang CT, ARCNET Research Group. Changing age distribution of the donor population in the United States. *Transfusion* 2007 Nov 13 [Epub ahead of print].

[21] Slichter SJ. Platelet transfusion therapy. *Haematol Oncol Clin North Am*. 2007 21(4): 697-729.

[22] Stroncek DF, Rebulla P. Platelet transfusion. *Lancet* 2007 370(9585:427-438.

[23]Carless PA, Rubens FD, Anthony DM, O'Connell D, Henry DA. Platelet-rich – plasmapheresis for minimizing peri-operative allogeneic blood transfusion. Cochranne *Database Syst Rev.* 2003;(2):CD004172.

[24]Valleley MS, Buckley KW, Hayes KM, Fortuna RR, Geiss DM, Holt DW. Are there benefits to fresh whole blood vs. packed red blood cell cardiopulmonary bypass prime on outcome in neonatal and pediatric cardiac surgery? *Extra Corpor Technol.* 2007 39(3):168-176.

[25]Hughes JD, Macdonald VW, Hess JR. Warm storage of whole blood for 72 hours. *Transfusion* 2007 47(11):2050-2056.

[26]Cobain TJ, Vamvakas EC, Wells A, Titlestad K. A survey of the demographics of blood use. *Transfusion Med.* 2007 (17): 1-15.

[27]Cameron B,Rock G, Olberg B, Neurath D. Evaluation of platelet transfusion triggers in a tertiary-care hospital. *Transfusion* 2007 47(2): 206-211.

[28]Greeno E, McCullough J, Weisdorf D. Platelet utilization and the transfusion trigger: a prospective analysis. *Transfusion* 2007 47(2):201-205.

[29]New HV. Paediatric transfusion. *Vox Sang.* 2006 90(10:1-9.

[30]Tinegate HN, Thompson CL, Jones H, Stainsby D. Where and when is blood transfused? An observational study of timing and location of red cell transfusions in north of England. *Vox Sang.* 2007 93(3):229-232.

[31]Eindhoven GB, Diercks RL, Richardson FJ, van Raaij JJ, Hagenaars JA, van Horn JR, de Wolf JT. Adjusted transfusion triggers improve transfusion practice in orthopaedic surgery. *Transfus Med.* 2005 15(1):13-18.

[32]Goodnough LT. Transfusion triggers. *Surgery* 2007 142(4 Suppl): S67-70.

[33]Moiz B, Arif FM, Hashmi KZ. Appropriate and inappropriate use of fresh frozen plasma. *J Pak Med Assoc.* 2006 56(8):356-359.

[34]Wallis JP, Wells AW, Chapman CE. Changing indications for red cell transfusion from 2000 to 2004 in the North of England. *Transfus Med.* 2006 16(6):411-417.

[35]Mueller MM, Seifried E. Blood transfusion in Europe: basic principles for initial and continuous training in transfusion medicine: an approach to a European harmonisation. *Tranfus Clin Biol.* 2006 13(5):282-285.

[36]Perez ER, Winters JL, Gajic O. The addition of decision support into computerized physician order entry reduces red blood cell transfusion resource utilization in the intensive care unit. *Am J Hematol.* 2007 82(7):631-633.

[37]Rana R, Afessa B, Keegan MT, Whalen FX Jr, Nuttall GA, Evenson LK, Peters SG, Winters JL, Hubmayr RD, Moore SB, Gajic O, Transfusion in the ICU Interest Group. Evidence-based red cell transfusion in the critically ill:quality improvement using computerized physician order entry. *Crit Care Med.* 2006 34(7):1892-1897.

[38]Gould S, Cimino MJ, Gerber DR. Packed red blood cell transfusion in the intensive care unit: limitations and consequences. *Am J Crit Care.* 2007 16(1):39-48.

[39]Rock G, Berger R, Filion D, Touche D, Neurath D, Wells G, Elsaadany S, Afzal M. Documenting a transfusion: how well is it done? *Transfusion* 2007 47(4):568-572.

[40]Shariff MM, Maqbool S, Butt TK, Iqbal S, Mumtaz A. Justifying the clinical use of fresh frozen plasma-an audit. *J Coll Physicians Surg Pak.* 2007 17(4):207-210.

[41]Fung MK, Downes KA, Shulman IA. Transfusion of platelets containing ABO-incompatible plasma: a survey of 3156 North American laboratories. *Arch Pathol Lab Med.* 2007 131(6):909-916.

[42]Ghigilone M. Blood Management: a model of excellence. *Clin Leadersh Manag Rev.* 2007 21(2): E2.

[43]Shander A, Goodnough LT. Update on transfusion medicine. *Pharmacotherapy* 2007 (9 Pt 2):57S-68S.

[44]Sagawa K. Guidelines for safer and more appropriate use of blood transfusion systems in Japan. *Nippon Geka Gakkai Zasshi.* 2005 106(1):7-12.

[45]Takahashi K. New guidelines for transfusion medicine. *Rinsho Byori.* 2006 54(12):1234-1240.

[46]O'Shaughnessy DF, Atterbury C, Bolton Maggs P, Murphy M, Thomas D, Yates S, Williamson LM, British Committee for Standards in Haematology, Blood Transfusion Task Force. Guidelines for the use of fresh-frozen plasma, cryoprecipitate and cryosupernatant. *Br J Haematol.* 2004 126(1):11-28.

[47]Buiting AM, van Aken WG. The practice guideline "Blood transfusion" (third integral revision). *Ned Tijdschr Geneeskd.* 2005 149(47):2613-2618.

[48]International Society of Blood Transfusion Information Security Task Force, Bobos A, Boecker W, Childers R, Couture A, Davis R, Espensen L, Fournier S, Holcombe J, Hulleman R, Lupo B, McDonnell S, Mokros I, Munk C, Steinke W, Wurzbach T. ISBT guidelines for information security in transfusion medicen. *Vox Sang.* 2006 Suppl 1: S1-S23.

[49]British Committee for Standards in Haematology, Stainsby D, MacLennan S, Thomas D, Isaac J, Hamilton PJ. Guidelines on the management of massive blood loss. *Br J Haematol.* 2006 135(5):634-641.

[50]Spiess BD. Red Cell transfusion and guidelines: a work in progress. *Hematol Oncol Clin North Am.* 2007 21(1):185-200.

[51]Bosly A, Muylle L, Noens L, Pietersz R, Heims D, Hubner R, Selleslag D, Toungouz M, Ferrant A, Sondag D. Guidelines for the transfusion of platelets. *Acta Clin Belg.* 2007 62(1):36-47.

[52]Society of Thoracic Surgeons Blood Conservation Guideline Task Force, Ferraris VA, Ferraris SP, Saha SP, Hessel EA 2nd, Haan CK, Royston BD, Bridges CR, Higgins RS, Despotis G, Brown JR, Society of Cardiovascular Anaesthesiologists Special Task Force on Blood Transfusion, Spiess BD, Shore-Lesserson L, Stafford-Smith M, Mazer CD, Bennett-Guerrero E, Hill SE, Body S. Perioperative blood transfusion and blood conservation in cardiac surgery: the Society of Thoracic Surgeons and The Society of Cardiovascular Anesthesiologists clinical practice guideline. *Am Thorac Surg.* 2007 83(5 Suppl):S27-S86.

[53]O'Riordan JM, Fitzgerald J, Smith OP, Bonnar J, Gorman WA, National Blood Users Group. Transfusion of blood components to infant under four months: review and guidelines. *Ir Med J.* 2007 100(6): suppl 1-24.

[54]Rebuck JA. Practical considerations when developing guidelines for managing critical bleeding. *Pharmacotherapy* 2007 27(9 pt 2): 103S-109S.

[55]Slichter SJ. Evidence-based platelet transfusion guidelines. *Hematology Am Soc Hematol Educ Program* 2007 2007:172-178.

[56]Transfusion Task Force. Amendments and corrections to the "Transfusion Guidelines for neonates and older children" (BCSH, 2004a); and to the "Guidelines for the use of fresh frozen plasma, cryoprecipitate and cryosupernatant" (BCSH, 2004b). *Br J Hematol* 2007 136(3):514-516.

[57]NHMRC/ASBT . Clinical Practice Guidelines on the Use of Blood Components (red blood cells, platelets, fresh frozen plasma, cryoprecipitate). Endorsed September 2001. Published by Commonwealth of Australia 2002.
[58]Cobain TJ. Fresh Blood Product Manufacture, Issue and Use: A Chain of Diminishing Returns? *Transfusion Medicine Reviews*. 2004 (18): 279- 292.

In: Transfusion - Think About It
Editor: Trevor J. Cobain
ISBN 978-1-61668-969-8

Chapter 5

BLOOD STORAGE LESIONS AND THEIR CLINICAL CONSEQUENCES

James P. Isbister
University of Sydney, New South Wales, Australia.

ABSTRACT

It is clearly established that blood is altered from the moment of collection. Anticoagulation, fractionation, cooling, preservation and storage time compound and progressively increase changes until the date of expiry [1,2]. The extent of these changes is determined by the collection technique, the specific blood component, the preservative medium, the container, storage time and storage conditions. The threshold storage time for blood components has generally been arbitrarily determined by *in vitro* studies and assessment of *in vivo* survival. In the case of red cell concentrates, greater than 75% of transfused cells should survive at 24 hours post-transfusion. As will be discussed there are no established clinical criteria for post-transfusion efficacy of red cell transfusions.

There is evidence to indicate that blood storage lesions are clinically significant and that these can be prevented or minimized by prestorage leucodepletion.

INTRODUCTION

There are many landmarks in the history of blood transfusion, but few rival the discovery by Landsteiner of the ABO blood groups followed by the development of methods for preserving and fractionating blood. In the early days, before blood could be anticoagulated or stored, direct donor vein to recipient vein was the usual practice (figure 1).

The patient thus received warm and fresh "unaltered" ABO compatible blood and storage lesions were not an issue. From the outset there would be clear advantages if firstly, the patient and the donor could be separated in place (by anticoagulation) and secondly, in time (by preservation). The introduction of citrate achieved the first, but cold storage was only possible for a few days and it was not until the introduction of ACD during WW2 that preservation became a reality. Interestingly, early last century, before preservatives were introduced there was debate regarding the advantages of defibrination of donor blood over citrate for maintaining blood fluidity prior to transfusion. Defibrination, although a more complex method, offered an advantage that the collected blood could be stored for longer periods of time. In retrospect this raises the possibility that the prestorage leucoreduction, inherent in the defibrination process improved the viability of red cells during storage (*vide infra*).

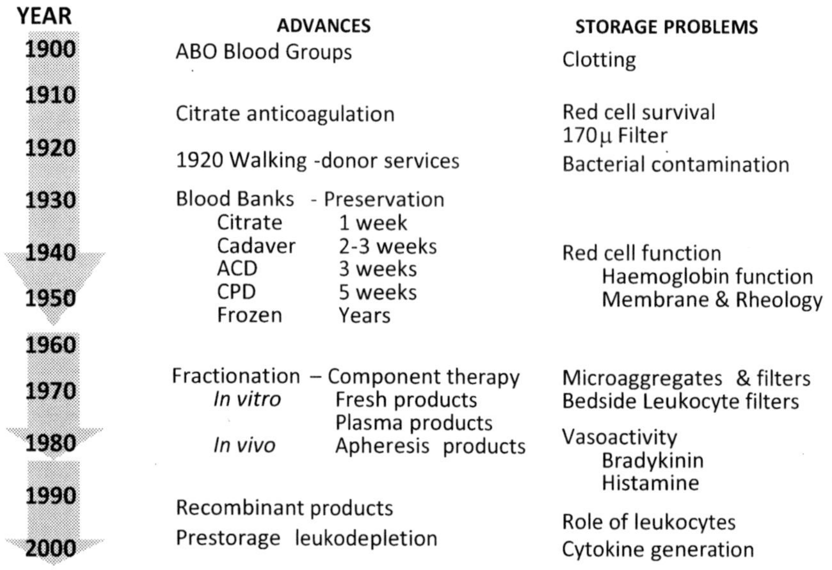

YEAR
ADVANCES
STORAGE PROBLEMS
1900
ABO Blood Groups
Clotting
1910
Citrate anticoagulation
Red cell survival
170μ Filter
1920
1920 Walking -donor services
Bacterial contamination
1930
Blood Banks - Preservation
Citrate 1 week
Cadaver 2-3 weeks
ACD 3 weeks
CPD 5 weeks
Frozen Years
1940
Red cell function
Haemoglobin function
Membrane & Rheology
1950
1960
Fractionation – Component therapy
In vitro Fresh products
Plasma products
In vivo Apheresis products
1970
Microaggregates & filters
Bedside Leukocyte filters
1980
Vasoactivity
Bradykinin
Histamine
1990
Recombinant products
Prestorage leukodepletion
2000
Role of leukocytes
Cytokine generation

Figure 1. Historical Milestones in Preservation & Storage of Blood.

Stored red cells have changes in their shape, deformability and haemoglobin function that, if the cells survive, may take several hours to return to normal post transfusion. Blood storage lesions impacting on the efficacy and safety of transfusion are most relevant in relationship to the labile blood components, especially the cellular components stored in the liquid state [3–7]. Red cell concentrates are the most widely used blood component in this respect. Platelet concentrates, with a much shorter storage time and the requirement that they be stored at 22-24°C, is a constant challenge for blood supply agencies and present additional problems, especially in relationship to bacterial contamination, activation and cytokine accumulation [8,9].

Most research focusing on the preparation, preservation and storage of blood components has been *in vitro,* with analysis carried out on biochemical parameters (e.g., ATP, pH, 2,3 DPG) and occasionally membrane, morphological and rheological characteristics [2,10-14] (figure 2).

In vivo studies have generally focused on intravascular survival of transfused blood components and, to a lesser extent, post-transfusion function, clinical efficacy and patient outcomes. In recent years more detailed attention is being given to assessing potential adverse clinical consequences of storage changes in the clinical use of blood components. Concern has been expressed by clinicians for decades in relationship to efficacy of stored fresh blood products and the potential for the storage lesion to have adverse impact of patient outcomes. It has been difficult to prove clinical efficacy and safety in prospective clinical studies due to the multifactorial nature and complexity of many transfusion settings, especially hemorrhagic shock and trauma. There is no question that transfusion of stored blood saves lives in the acute haemorrhagic and critical anaemia settings and randomised clinical trials will probably never be carried out comparing ultra fresh blood transfusion with that of stored blood transfusion in relationship to better clinical outcomes.

Quantitative deficiency

1. Pre/post transfusion red cell death
2. Failure to achieve anticipated end points
3. Excessive donor exposure to achieve efficacy
   - Transfusion related infections
   - Greater exposure to alloimmunsation

Qualitative deficiency

1. Decreased membrane flexibility and increased adhesion to endothelium → impaired microcirculatory haemodynamics
2. Reduced 2,3 DPG
   → Hb affinity O_2↑ → ?Impaired O_2 unloading
   → Depleted Nitric Oxide → ?Impair microcirculatory regulation

Figure 2. The impact of storage on red cell and haemoglobin function.

There is always a heated debate when the use of fresh blood is discussed as it is sometimes viewed as an anathema to the philosophy of blood banking. The focused clinician, confronted with a critically bleeding patient, may state: *"My patient bleeds fresh whole blood, therefore, he needs fresh whole blood."* In contrast blood bankers promote the concept that the mix of stored red cells, platelet concentrates, factor concentrates and fresh frozen plasma is equivalent to fresh whole blood. Blood bankers advocate that haemopoietic defects should be identified by laboratory testing and corrected with specific blood components as indicated. A pre-emptive approach to the prevention of defects has generally been discouraged. However, there is no doubt that there are significant implications relating to storage (figure 3).

Ironically, if stored whole blood was today submitted as a new therapeutic to regulatory authorities for registration, one suspects there would be requirements that initial clinical studies should use fresh blood to demonstrate efficacy and safety. Following such evidence, consideration for extending the shelf-life could be submitted. The fact that the debate regarding the advantages of fresh whole blood continues highlights the fact that we do not have a definitive answer. When one is unable to prove, in a truly scientific manner and based on clinical trials, that a form of therapy is efficacious or not, one has to fall back on a sound logical use of the currently available scientific understanding.

Quality and safety in transfusion medicine has predominantly focused on the well understood and reported hazards of transfusion, the immunological, technical and infectious. These are generally unifactorial with a 1:1 causal relationship between the blood component transfused, usually a specific individual unit, and the adverse consequence for the patient. Blood group incompatibility (especially ABO), transfusion related infection transmission (HIV and hepatitis), transfusion associated graft versus host disease (TAGVHD) are in this category. These are transfusion complications in which the cause can be clearly established and in most cases prevented.

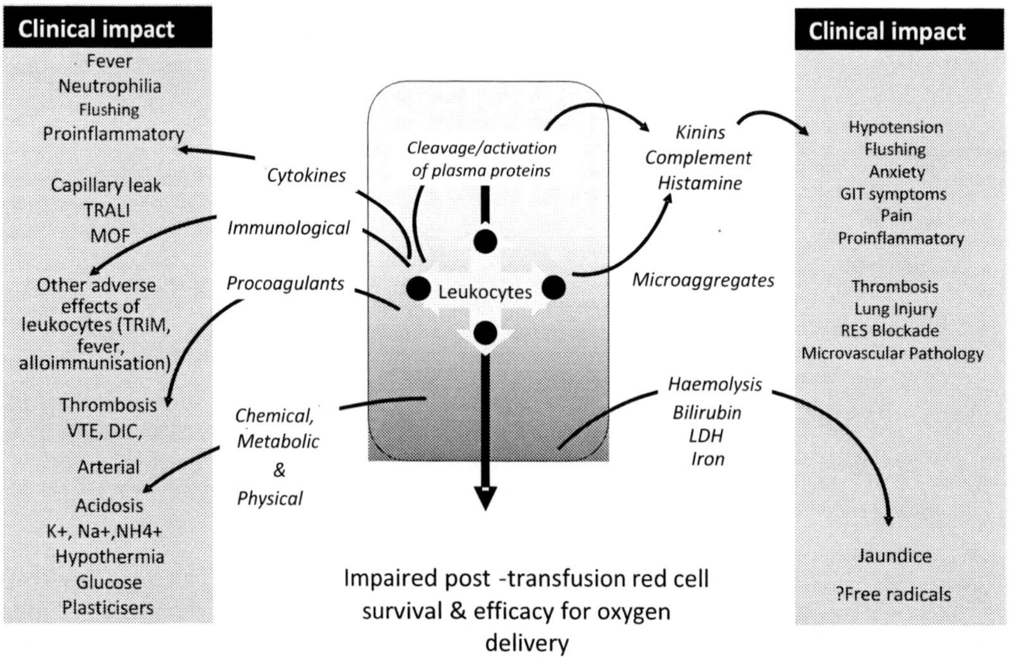

Figure 3. Whole blood storage lesions and the clinical impacts.

In contrast there are many adverse effects of transfusion in which causation may be more difficult to establish. However, there is increasing evidence that some adverse consequences of transfusion result from interaction with other insults, pathophysiology or host factors, in which the contribution of the transfusion can usually be specifically identified. Fever, allergic reactions, hypotensive reactions, transfusion related circulatory overload (TACO), some cases of transfusion related acute lung injury (TRALI), hyperbilirubinaemia and CMV transmission are examples of this category.

With these established potential hazards of allogeneic blood transfusion, greater attention is now being given to the issue of transfusion and its relationship to adverse clinical outcomes. The functional quality and post-transfusion efficacy of labile blood components is receiving closer attention. Allogeneic transfusion is being associated with increased morbidity, mortality (sepsis, lung injury and multi-organ failure) and prolongation of ICU and/or length of hospital stay. It is difficult to implicate transfusion directly in an individual case, but strong association has been established in numerous observational studies, but causation can only be confidently identified by large, well-conducted randomised controlled trials. Accumulating evidence, in the absence of such trials, supports causation thus demanding a more precautionary approach to allogeneic blood transfusion, examination of alternatives to transfusion and implementation of methods to improve the quality of transfused labile blood components. The underlying pathophysiology of these adverse outcomes probably relates to transfusion-induced immunomodulation (TRIM) causing immunosuppression and the storage lesions. Universal pre-storage leucodepletion is currently the most important and effective strategy for minimizing the clinical impacts of TRIM and the storage lesion [15-18]. Parallel to this epidemiological evidence there is a wealth of supporting *in vitro* data and animal studies raising concerns that the changes resulting from storage of blood components may have adverse clinical consequences [19].

Resulting from these broader concerns about the efficacy and safety of allogeneic blood transfusion, more attention is being directed towards questions of transfusion appropriateness, the quality of blood products and the clinical consequences of transfusion-related immunomodulation (TRIM), blood storage lesions, bacterial contamination and transfusion related acute lung injury (TRALI) [20-30].

Blood Storage Lesions

Blood storage may result in quantitative and/or qualitative deficiencies in blood components that may thus jeopardise the efficacy and safety of a transfusion [31,32]. Parallel with these storage changes there is an accumulation of degenerate material (e.g., microaggregates and procoagulant material), release of vasoactive agents, cytokine generation, and haemolysis [16,17,18]. Many of the changes occurring during storage are related to the presence of leucocytes and can be minimised by pre-storage leukoreduction [16]. During storage red cells undergo a change from their "resting" state as a biconcave disc shape to cells with spiky projections termed echinocytes, eventually becoming sphereo-echinocytes with impaired cellular deformability [19,31]. Blood is a thyxotropic fluid (Non Newtonian fluid) increasing its fluidity the higher the shear rate. This characteristic of blood and the ability of red cells to traverse capillaries is dependent on red cell flexibility. Red cell membrane changes with storage also increase their tendency to adhere to endothelial cell surfaces in the microcirculation, especially if there is any activation of endothelial cells such as may occur in the presence of the systemic inflammatory response (e.g., secondary to shock or sepsis) [33]. With these membrane changes there is an accumulation of the microvesicles that may be thrombogenic [34-37].

There is accumulating evidence that the immediate post-transfusion function of stored red cells and haemoglobin in delivering and unloading oxygen to the microcirculation is questionable and several hours are required for red cell oxygen carriage and delivery return to normal [38,39]. The role of red cells and haemoglobin in microvascular blood flow control has been receiving considerable attention in recent years [40,41]. Nitric oxide has a fundamental role in maintaining and controlling microvascular vasomotor tone with haemoglobin and red cells having a critical role in regulating the activity of nitric oxide in the vascular compartment. It is thus not surprising that there is now interest in how the storage of red cells may impact on their post-transfusion function in this respect [42]. There is recent evidence that red cell storage results in depletion of nitric oxide compromising red cell induced microcirculatory vasodilatory response to hypoxia. It has been demonstrated that S-nitrosohemoglobin concentrations decline rapidly on storage and hypoxic vasodilation by banked RBCs correlates with the S-nitrosohemoglobin levels. Reconstitution of S-nitrosohemoglobin levels in stored blood in an animal model restored vasodilatory activity [43-45].

There is also *in vivo* evidence in hamsters that stored red cells are effective in reconstituting the macrocirculation and that benefit at a microcirculatory level is secondary to this systemic effect. Exchange transfusion with 28-day stored red cells versus fresh red cells impaired microvascular perfusion, yet differences at the systemic level were not apparent. The principal differences between fresh and stored red cells at the microvascular level were reduction in the functional capillary density and blood flow [46].

Clinical Significance of Storage Lesions of Red Cell Concentrates

The clinical significance of blood storage lesions is a matter of heated debate; in some cases adverse effects are widely accepted, while in others further studies are needed [47].

Evidence includes:

- Transfusion of red cell concentrates for clinically stable patients in the critical care setting to achieve a haemoglobin level >80gm/L does not improve outcome and may indeed be detrimental [48,49].
- It has been difficult to confirm the benefit of red cell transfusions in the peri-operative period and there is no agreement as to the haemoglobin level at which outcome is improved by transfusion [49].
- Benchmarking studies demonstrate considerable differences in transfusion practices between individual hospitals and clinicians [50].
- In years past the mortality of trauma patients requiring massive transfusions of >20 units of blood declined dramatically [51]. Almost 50% of trauma patients requiring >50 units of blood are surviving, but there is disturbing evidence, on the basis of observational studies, that the transfusions are an independent risk factor for poorer survival, increased infection rates, prolongation of length of hospital stay and development of the multi-organ failure syndrome and adult respiratory distress syndrome.
- The transfusion of stored red cells in the bleeding setting are effective in restoring the macrocirculation, but are less effective in the microcirculation and may be detrimental to microcirculatory function [46,52].

Observational studies demonstrate that red cell transfusions may be an additional risk factor for such conditions as adult respiratory distress syndrome (ARDS), multi-organ failure (MOF), vasoactive reactions and alterations in laboratory parameters (table 1) [38,53-57].

It is assumed that blood components have been appropriately collected, processed, stored, transported and transfused. Although there is now closer attention to standard operating procedures and regulations that apply to these aspects of the blood component supply chain, quality of the final product cannot be guaranteed [58]. The "assumed" quality of labile cellular blood products is based on research data and monitoring of standard operative procedures. There is no red cell blood product assessment prior to transfusion [39]. It is, however, generally accepted that the adverse effects of storage increase with time and an arbitrary "cut off" is mandated on the basis of research studies.

Table 1. The red cell storage lesion and the possible clinical consequences

Storage lesion	Potential Clinical Consequence/s
Alterations in red cell structure & function	
ATP Depletion	Echino-spherocyte formation, increased osmotic fragility, impaired red cell deformability with adverse effects on O_2 transport and delivery
Microvesiculation and loss of membrane lipid, lipid peroxidation and haemolysis and irreversible damaged red cells	Reduced red cell viability and cell death Hyperbilirubinaemia, LDH, increased serum Iron ?free radical generation, hyperkalaemia
Reduced 2, 3 DPG	Increased haemoglobin affinity for O_2 and impaired unloading
Decreased CD47 antigen (integrin-associated protein) expression	Reduced post-transfusion survival due to premature clearance post-transfusion
Red cell adhesion to endothelial cells	Adverse effects on the microcirculatory haemodynamics
Depletion of Nitric Oxide	?Impair microcirculatory regulation
Storage temperature	Hypothermia unless pretransfusion warming
Additives	
Citrate	Hypocalcaemia, Acid-base imbalance Initial acidosis > alkalosis
Glucose	Hyperglycaemia
Sodium	Hypernatraemia
Accumulants	
Cytokines: IL-1,IL-6,IL-8,TNF-α	Fever, hypotension, flushing
Enzymes: myeloperoxidase, elastase, arginase, secretory phospholipase A_2,	Transfusion related Immunomodulation (TRIM) Neutrophilia
Reactive proteins: defensins, annexin, soluble HLA, FasLigand, soluble endothelial cell growth factor and others	Proinflammatory with potentiation of SIRS Potential "priming" for ARDS, TRALI and MODS Hypotension, anxiety, flushing, pain syndromes, proinflammatory
Histamine and kinin accumulation	Blockade of reticuloendothelial system
Microaggregates, microvesiculation and accumulation of procoagulants	Risk factor for development of acute lung injury and MOF Activation of haemostasis > ?DIC ?VTE ?arterial thrombotic events

Possible mechanisms and potential clinical consequences of the storage lesion includes:-

Quantitative and qualitative deficiency of blood components

- Failure to achieve anticipated end points, real or surrogate, due to reduced quantity and/or functional quality of the blood product.
- As a result of reduced post-transfusion survival there may be exposure to excessive numbers of donors to achieve the anticipated end point.

Physical characteristics

- Hypothermia

Chemical characteristics

- Citrate toxicity [59]
- Electrolyte and Acid-base imbalance [60]
- Glucose loads

Contamination

- Bacterial contamination resulting in endotoxaemia or septicaemia [61]
- Plasticisers [62]

Accumulation of "toxic" or degenerate products

- Role of the storage lesion in transfusion related immunomodulation [63]
    - Role of cytokines [64,65]
    - Role of reticuloendothelial system blockade
- Accentuation of free radical pathophysiology due to hyperferraemia [66]
- Effects of transfusion on laboratory parameters (e.g., hyperbilirubinaemia, neutrophilia, hyperferraemia and elevated lactic dehydrogenase) that may result in incorrect interpretation [67,68]
- a risk factor for multi-organ failure (MOF) and adult respiratory distress syndrome (ARDS) [69,70]
- Early hyperkalaemia, hypocalcaemia [71-73]
- Activation and consumption of the haemostatic factors with possible contribution to coagulopathy and venous thromboembolism [74,75]
- Non haemolytic, non-febrile transfusion reactions [76,77]
- Hypotension and circulatory instability due to vasoactive substance (kinins, histamine) [57,78].

The Association of Allogeneic Transfusion with Poorer Clinical Outcomes

Observational clinical studies have identified blood transfusion as a possible independent risk factor for morbidity and mortality and increased length of hospital stay and additional costs [21,79,80]. In particular, TRALI is receiving attention as a potentially serious complication of blood transfusion [22,23,81,82]. In the classical plasma-neutrophil-antibody mediated form of this complication, symptoms arise within hours of a blood transfusion [83,84]. The underlying pathophysiology of "classical" TRALI is due to the presence of leucoagglutinins in donor plasma, usually from multiparous female donors. When complement is activated, C5a promotes granulocyte aggregation and sequestration in the microcirculation of the lung leading to endothelial damage and interstitial oedema, proceeding onto acute respiratory failure. It is now recognised that there has been under-recognition and under-diagnosis of TRALI, partly due to a lack of clinical awareness, but also a lack of a broader understanding of potential mechanisms by which blood transfusion may cause or be a contributory factor to lung injury [85-88]. The term TRALI is now being expanded beyond those cases due to anti-neutrophil antibodies to consider cases in which transfusion is identified as an independent risk factor predisposing patients to lung injury [89]. There are several recent reviews addressing this expanding area of concern in which transfusion *per se* is being identified as an independent risk factor for poor clinical poor outcomes, of which TRALI is only one [81,88,90-92].

Blood transfusion being implicated as part of the problem rather than optimal therapy has been a surprise to many clinicians, as it has always been assumed that blood transfusion can only be of benefit to the bleeding or anaemic patient. These concerns are resulting in reassessment of management of critical haemorrhage and anaemia and challenging of longstanding dogmas [93-96]. There is greater tolerance of hypotension until haemorrhage is controlled, lower haemoglobin levels are tolerated with closer attention to the clinical context of the anaemia and its impact on systemic and local oxygen delivery, especially if there are compromises in cardiorespiratory function. The evidence that the immediate post-transfusion ability of stored red cells and haemoglobin to deliver and unload oxygen to microcirculation may be impaired is challenging the long held view that stored red cell concentrates should automatically be the first therapy for acutely enhancing oxygen delivery. More attention and research is focusing on the composition of clear fluids, the importance of plasma viscosity, colloid oncotic pressure and functional capillary density [97-103]. Along with this is development of the concept of targeted oxygen therapy with high inspired oxygen levels, hyperbaric oxygen and a re-evaluation of haemoglobin based oxygen carriers [104-109].

There are thus many questions being asked about the safety and efficacy of allogeneic blood transfusion and the possibility/probability that transfusion may not only be part of the solution, but be partly responsible for poorer clinical outcomes. Having recognised and acknowledged these concerns it is important to emphasise that transfusion of the critically haemorrhaging patient can be life saving, but the quality and quantity of the transfused blood component is important.

In recent years there has been a reassessment of the management of the acutely haemorrhaging patient. Advances in patient retrieval, resuscitation protocols, techniques for rapid and real time diagnosis, trauma teams and early "damage control" surgery have all improved the management of acutely haemorrhaging patients [110]. Patients are now surviving with larger volumes of blood transfusion, but sepsis, acute lung injury and multi-organ failure remain major challenges and blood transfusion is increasingly being recognised as a two-edged sword and probably a contributory factor to these complications in which microcirculatory dysfunction is recognised as central in the pathophysiology [51]. Observational studies have identified blood transfusion as an independent risk factor for morbidity and mortality [80,111-114]. Correlation does not mean causation, but on critical assessment of the evidence, it is likely to be the case. This has lead to a re-analysis of guidelines for the management of acutely bleeding patients. Clinical practice guidelines should no longer primarily address the management of massive blood transfusion, but rather the management of critical bleeding and quality/efficacy of blood components. The *modus operandi* is now pre-emptive, instituting measures to avoid getting into the massive transfusion and coagulopathy quagmire in which the patient spirals down into the "triad of death": coagulopathy, acidosis and hypothermia. Stored red cells are pro-inflammatory and procoagulant [16,75,115-117].

Does the Storage Age of Blood Matter?

Similar to the ultra fresh blood controversy there is an ongoing debate as to the difference between "young" stored blood and "old" stored blood with equally vocal proponents at each end of the spectrum [118,119]. There is general acceptance that from *in vitro* and some animal *in vivo* evidence that stored blood deteriorates over time and must have a use by date [32,120]. The controversy centres around the clinical significance of storage age and patient clinical outcomes [42,54,121-124]. However, as the evidence and literature on this topic accumulates, albeit conflicting, it is the author's view that the ageing of stored blood is clinically significant [68]. The Canadian clinical trials group are initiating a randomised controlled trial addressing this question as there are major implications for blood supply agencies and the quality of stored blood components [125]. Interest has recently been stimulated by a retrospective observational study in cardiac surgery patients, suggesting increased morbidity and mortality in patients receiving red cell transfusion more than 14 days old [126]. A study in patients with severe traumatic brain injury and other trauma patients raises similar concerns [121,127]. There has also been and extensive literature and conflicting evidence associating allogeneic blood transfusion cancer recurrence rates [128]. This issue is not reviewed in this chapter, however, there is evidence that if there is a causal relationship that transfusion related immunomodulation may not be the only mechanism responsible and the storage lesion *per se* may have a role [63]. A recent study in rates with autologous blood in this regard is particularly provocative and supports the observational evidence that transfusion should be avoided/minimised in cancer surgery as a precautionary measure [129,130].

Taking a precautionary approach it is probably reasonable to state that significant changes occur in non leucoreduced red cell concentrates after 14 days storage that may be clinical significant. There is insufficient evidence to know to what degree the red cell storage lesion is minimised by the buffy coat removal in the preparation of platelet concentrates and/or pre-storage leucodepletion. In determining priority for fresher red cell concentrates the volume, rate, frequency of infusion and clinical condition of the patient need to be considered. Neonates, especially exchange transfusion, massive blood transfusion and patients with cardiorespiratory impairment warrant attention to the age of blood for transfusion.

In regard to platelet concentrates the issues are more complex as the actual mechanisms by which stored platelets are haemostatic are controversial as platelet microparticles formed during storage may be the main haemostatic component until stored platelet function returns to normal post-transfusion [131].

PREVENTION AND/OR MINIMISATION OF THE STORAGE LESION AND ITS CLINICAL CONSEQUENCES

Accepting that that blood storage lesions are clinically significant it is important to differentiate between storage lesions being responsible for failure to achieve clinical/laboratory endpoints as a result of reduced survival and/or qualitative defects in cellular function, and the "toxic" effects of storage. Clearly, avoiding or minimising the use of allogeneic blood transfusions by appropriate clinical decision making and use of alternatives is self evident in order to reduce the clinical impact of storage lesions [132-134].

Several approaches are available to prevent or minimise the red cell storage lesion and its clinical consequences (figure 4).

Blood supply agencies in developed countries are generally externally regulated and have standard operating procedures stemming from long established and tested methods for the collection and preservation of labile blood components. There are continuing efforts to improve blood preservation with the aim of supplying better quality products [58]. At present however, assuming integrity of the current processes, pre-storage leucoreduction to <1 x 10^6/L is probably the most effective intervention to improve the post-transfusion survival and quality of red cell and platelet concentrates [135-143]. Cellular blood products contain variable numbers of donor leucocytes that are essentially contaminants responsible for undesirable and potentially hazardous consequence of blood component therapy. Other than the storage lesions leucoreduction has been proven to be of importance in preventing or minimising several adverse effects of allogeneic blood transfusion [144]. Leucoreduction has long been advocated to reduce the incidence and/or delay the onset of alloimmunisation to leucocytes with the aim of preventing non-haemolytic febrile transfusion reactions, minimising the development of refractoriness to platelet transfusions, and improving access to potential donors for tissue transplantation. Leucocytes also act as the principal reservoirs and/or transport vehicles for a range of cell associated viral, bacterial and protozoal pathogens. Evidence also supports a protective role for leucocyte-depletion against a range of transfusion transmitted infections especially CMV.

1. Avoid or minimise transfusion
   - Clinical practice guidelines
   - Tolerance of anaemia
   - Optimizing red cell mass
   - Minimise blood loss
   - Use of alternatives
2. As far as possible use "freshest" blood products
   - Prioritise patients
     - Neonates, massive transfusion, cardiorespiratory compromise
3. Minimise the storage lesion
   - Collection methods and preservation solutions
   - SOPs and Quality control
   - Universal prestorage leucoreduction
4. Minimise the clinical consequences of the storage lesion
   - Premedication and rate of transfusion
   - Minimise transfusion volume
   - Identify high risk patients
   - Awareness of potential clinical effects of storage lesions
   - Early recognition, correct diagnosis and management of adverse clinical events that may be related to the storage lesions

Figure 4. Prevention and minimisation of the storage lesion and its clinical consequences.

Recent studies have identified that there are questions about the role of red cell transfusions in many clinical settings and dogmas about the appropriateness of red cell transfusion are being questioned. The benefits of transfusion have been assumed in many clinical circumstance and it is a sobering thought to consider that when there is questionable evidence for benefit from blood transfusion a patient may be unnecessarily exposed to potential morbidity or mortality. There is no denying the decision-making for blood component therapy can be difficult and much debate continues in relation to the indications for the use of various blood components [132]. However, there are good common sense and scientifically evidence-based reasons to adopt a non-transfusion default position when there is poor evidence for potential benefit. Clearly, if allogeneic blood component therapy can be avoided the potential hazards need not be considered and storage age becomes irrelevant.

Conclusion

There is now evidence that blood storage lesions are clinically significant. It is important to differentiate between the storage lesion that is responsible for failure to achieve clinical/laboratory endpoints: reduced survival, qualitative defects in cellular function, and the "toxic" effects of storage. Applying the precautionary principle, it is reasonable to conclude that in the case of red cell concentrates, significant changes occur in non leucoreduced products after 7-10 days. As leucocytes are largely responsible for the clinically significant storage changes, the wider use of universal pre-storage leucoreduction minimises the problem.

Blood filters have always been a subject of debate in transfusion medicine. The use of blood filters, whatever type, is an acknowledgement of the existence of the blood storage lesion and its probable clinical significance. The 170 μm filters in standard blood sets were originally introduced into transfusion medicine to prevent blood sets obstructing, not because of a concern that the fibrin clots may harm the patient. Fortunately the human lung is one of Nature's remarkable filters and receives all intravenous infusions on their "first pass". One presumes it was concluded, by trial and error, that 170 μm filters seemed to be the best compromise between using a larger needle and keeping the blood transfusion flowing. In the 1960's and 1970's interest arose in adult respiratory distress syndrome, mainly stimulated by experiences during the Vietnam War. Logic and animal data suggested that the unfiltered microaggregates accumulating during storage may be a contributor to the development of ARDS, and that microfilters to remove microparticles 20-40 μm in size may be protective [145-147]. Unfortunately, it was difficult to prove these in clinical trials for several reasons, especially the multifactorial nature of the clinical problem of massive blood transfusion and the less-sophisticated statistical methods than are currently available. Nevertheless, microaggregate filters are inadequate to significantly address the problem of the storage lesion and its clinical significance.

Preventing the development of the storage lesion from its inception, using pre-storage leucodepletion filters, is a more logical and scientific approach to the problem. The storage lesions of the commonly used labile blood components (i.e., red cell and platelet concentrates) and the clinical consequences, especially in the critical bleeding setting, are now receiving appropriate attention. Universal pre-storage leucoreduction is now standard practice in many countries. Ironically, its introduction was for other reasons than minimising the storage lesions, preventing leucocyte immunisation and immunomodulation and not on sound scientific evidence. Rather, they were introduced as a precautionary measure against the possible transfusion transmission of vCJD that subsequently turned out to be justified [148,149].

REFERENCES

[1] Valeri CR, Ragno G. Cryopreservation of human blood products. *Transfus Apher Sci* 2006.

[2] Scott KL, Lecak J, Acker JP. Biopreservation of red blood cells: past, present, and future. *Transfusion medicine reviews* 2005;19(2):127-42.

[3] Longster GH, Buckley T, Sikorski J, Derrick Tovey LA. Scanning electron microscope studies of red cell morphology. Changes occurring in red cell shape during storage and post transfusion. *Vox sanguinis* 1972;22(2):161-70.

[4] Solheim BG, Flesland O, Seghatchian J, Brosstad F. Clinical implications of red blood cell and platelet storage lesions: an overview. *Transfus Apheresis Sci* 2004;31(3):185-9.

[5] Hogman CF, Meryman HT. Storage parameters affecting red blood cell survival and function after transfusion. *Transfusion medicine reviews* 1999;13(4):275-96.

[6] Hogman CF. Liquid-stored red blood cells for transfusion. A status report. *Vox sanguinis* 1999;76(2):67-77.

[7] Hogman CF. Storage of blood components. *Current opinion in hematology* 1999;6(6):427-31.

[8] Yomtovian R. Bacterial contamination of blood: lessons from the past and road map for the future. *Transfusion* 2004;44(3):450-60.

[9] Heddle NM, Klama L, Meyer R, et al. A randomized controlled trial comparing plasma removal with white cell reduction to prevent reactions to platelets. *Transfusion* 1999;39(3):231-8.

[10] Schrier SL, Hardy B, Bensch K, Junga I, Krueger J. Red blood cell membrane storage lesion. *Transfusion* 1979;19(2):158-65.

[11] McCue JP, Vincent JM. Changes in red blood cell membrane phosphate concentration during blood bank storage. *Transfusion* 1981;21(1):107-12.

[12] Schrier SL, Sohmer PR, Moore GL, Ma L, Junga I. Red blood cell membrane abnormalities during storage: correlation with in vivo survival. *Transfusion* 1982;22(4):261-5.

[13] Dawson RB. Preservation of red blood cells for transfusion. *Human pathology* 1983;14(3):213-7.

[14] Hess JR. An update on solutions for red cell storage. *Vox sanguinis* 2006;91(1):13-9.

[15] Blumberg N, Heal JM. Universal leukocyte reduction of blood transfusions. *Clin Infect Dis* 2007;45(8):1014-5.

[16] Sparrow RL, Patton KA. Supernatant from stored red blood cell primes inflammatory cells: influence of prestorage white cell reduction. *Transfusion* 2004;44(5):722-30.

[17] Sparrow RL, Healey G, Patton KA, Veale MF. Red blood cell age determines the impact of storage and leukocyte burden on cell adhesion molecules, glycophorin A and the release of annexin V. *Transfus Apher Sci* 2006;34(1):15-23.

[18] Anniss AM, Glenister KM, Killian JJ, Sparrow RL. Proteomic analysis of supernatants of stored red blood cell products. *Transfusion* 2005;45(9):1426-33.

[19] Relevy H, Koshkaryev A, Manny N, Yedgar S, Barshtein G. Blood banking-induced alteration of red blood cell flow properties. *Transfusion* 2008;48(1):136-46.

[20] Wallis JP. Transfusion-related acute lung injury (TRALI)--under-diagnosed and under-reported. *British journal of anaesthesia* 2003;90(5):573-6.

[21] Shander A. Emerging risks and outcomes of blood transfusion in surgery. *Seminars in hematology* 2004;41(1 Suppl 1):117-24.
[22] Swanson K, Dwyre DM, Krochmal J, Raife TJ. Transfusion-related acute lung injury (TRALI): current clinical and pathophysiologic considerations. *Lung* 2006;184(3):177-85.
[23] Popovsky MA. Pulmonary consequences of transfusion: TRALI and TACO. *Transfus Apher Sci* 2006.
[24] Moore SB. Transfusion-related acute lung injury (TRALI): clinical presentation, treatment, and prognosis. *Critical care medicine* 2006;34(5 Suppl):S114-7.
[25] Blajchman MA. Immunomodulation and blood transfusion. *American journal of therapeutics* 2002;9(5):389-95.
[26] Raghavan M, Marik PE. Anemia, allogenic blood transfusion, and immunomodulation in the critically ill. *Chest* 2005;127(1):295-307.
[27] Mincheff MS, Meryman HT. Blood transfusion, blood storage and immunomodulation. *Immunol Invest* 1995;24(1-2):303-9.
[28] Pattison JW. Ensuring appropriate use of blood transfusion in anaemia. *Nursing times* 2005;101(15):30-3.
[29] Shander A, Goodnough LT. Objectives and limitations of bloodless medical care. *Current opinion in hematology* 2006;13(6):462-70.
[30] Hendrickson JE, Hillyer CD. Noninfectious serious hazards of transfusion. *Anesthesia and analgesia* 2009;108(3):759-69.
[31] Bosman GJ, Werre JM, Willekens FL, Novotny VM. Erythrocyte ageing in vivo and in vitro: structural aspects and implications for transfusion. *Transfusion medicine (Oxford, England)* 2008;18(6):335-47.
[32] Almac E, Ince C. The impact of storage on red cell function in blood transfusion. *Best Pract Res Clin Anaesthesiol* 2007;21(2):195-208.
[33] Anniss AM, Sparrow RL. Storage duration and white blood cell content of red blood cell (RBC) products increases adhesion of stored RBCs to endothelium under flow conditions. *Transfusion* 2006;46(9):1561-7.
[34] Kriebardis AG, Antonelou MH, Stamoulis KE, Economou-Petersen E, Margaritis LH, Papassideri IS. RBC-derived vesicles during storage: ultrastructure, protein composition, oxidation, and signaling components. *Transfusion* 2008;48(9):1943-53.
[35] Krailadsiri P, Seghatchian J, Macgregor I, et al. The effects of leukodepletion on the generation and removal of microvesicles and prion protein in blood components. *Transfusion* 2006;46(3):407-17.
[36] Salzer U, Zhu R, Luten M, et al. Vesicles generated during storage of red cells are rich in the lipid raft marker stomatin. *Transfusion* 2008;48(3):451-62.
[37] Greenwalt TJ. The how and why of exocytic vesicles. *Transfusion* 2006;46(1):143-52.
[38] Tinmouth A, Fergusson D, Yee IC, Hebert PC. Clinical consequences of red cell storage in the critically ill. *Transfusion* 2006;46(11):2014-27.
[39] Elfath MD. Is it time to focus on preserving the functionality of red blood cells during storage? *Transfusion* 2006;46(9):1469-70.
[40] Gladwin MT, Crawford JH, Patel RP. The biochemistry of nitric oxide, nitrite, and hemoglobin: role in blood flow regulation. *Free radical biology & medicine* 2004;36(6):707-17.

[41] Singel DJ, Stamler JS. Chemical physiology of blood flow regulation by red blood cells: the role of nitric oxide and S-nitrosohemoglobin. *Annual review of physiology* 2005;67:99-145.
[42] Raat NJ, Ince C. Oxygenating the microcirculation: the perspective from blood transfusion and blood storage. *Vox sanguinis* 2007;93(1):12-8.
[43] Bonaventura J. Clinical implications of the loss of vasoactive nitric oxide during red blood cell storage. *Proceedings of the National Academy of Sciences of the United States of America* 2007.
[44] Reynolds J, Ahearn G, Angelo M, Zhang J, Cobb F, Stamler J. S-nitrosohemoglobin deficiency: A mechanism for loss of physiological activity in banked blood. *PNAS* 2007;104(43):17058-0762.
[45] Winslow RM, Intaglietta M. Red cell age and loss of function: advance or SNO-job? *Transfusion* 2008;48(3):411-4.
[46] Tsai AG, Cabrales P, Intaglietta M. Microvascular perfusion upon exchange transfusion with stored red blood cells in normovolemic anemic conditions. *Transfusion* 2004;44(11):1626-34.
[47] Zimrin AB, Hess JR. Current issues relating to the transfusion of stored red blood cells. *Vox sanguinis* 2009;96(2):93-103.
[48] Hebert PC, Wells G, Blajchman MA, et al. A multicenter, randomized, controlled clinical trial of transfusion requirements in critical care. Transfusion Requirements in Critical Care Investigators, Canadian Critical Care Trials Group. *The New England journal of medicine* 1999;340(6):409-17.
[49] Carson JL, Hill S, Carless P, Hebert P, Henry D. Transfusion triggers: a systematic review of the literature. *Transfusion medicine reviews* 2002;16(3):187-99.
[50] Gombotz H, Rehak P, Shander A, Hofmann A. Blood use in elective surgery: the Austrian benchmark study. *Transfusion* 2007;47(8):1468-80.
[51] Hakala P, Hiippala S, Syrjala M, Randell T. Massive blood transfusion exceeding 50 units of plasma poor red cells or whole blood: the survival rate and the occurrence of leukopenia and acidosis. *Injury* 1999;30(9):619-22.
[52] Arslan E, Sierko E, Waters JH, Siemionow M. Microcirculatory hemodynamics after acute blood loss followed by fresh and banked blood transfusion. *American journal of surgery* 2005;190(3):456-62.
[53] Isbister JP. Is the clinical significance of blood storage lesions underestimated? *Trans Altern Trans Med* 2003;5(3):356-62.
[54] Basran S, Frumento RJ, Cohen A, et al. The association between duration of storage of transfused red blood cells and morbidity and mortality after reoperative cardiac surgery. *Anesthesia and analgesia* 2006;103(1):15-20, table of contents.
[55] Ho J, Sibbald WJ, Chin-Yee IH. Effects of storage on efficacy of red cell transfusion: when is it not safe? *Critical care medicine* 2003;31(12 Suppl):S687-97.
[56] Eastlund T. Vasoactive mediators and hypotensive transfusion reactions. *Transfusion* 2007;47(3):369-72.
[57] Isbister JP, Biggs JC. Reactions to rapid infusion of stable plasma protein solution during large volume plasma exchange. *Anaesthesia and intensive care* 1976;4(2):105-7.
[58] Hogman CF, Meryman HT. Red blood cells intended for transfusion: quality criteria revisited. *Transfusion* 2006;46(1):137-42.

[59] Dzik WH, Kirkley SA. Citrate toxicity during massive blood transfusion. *Transfusion medicine reviews* 1988;2(2):76-94.

[60] Wilson RF, Binkley LE, Sabo FM, Jr., et al. Electrolyte and acid-base changes with massive blood transfusions. *The American surgeon* 1992;58(9):535-44; discussion 44-5.

[61] Wagner SJ. Transfusion-transmitted bacterial infection: risks, sources and interventions. *Vox sanguinis* 2004;86(3):157-63.

[62] Baker RW. Diethylhexyl phthalate as a factor in blood transfusion and haemodialysis. *Toxicology* 1978;9(4):319-29.

[63] Vamvakas EC, Blajchman MA. Transfusion-related immunomodulation (TRIM): An update. *Blood reviews* 2007;21(6):327-48.

[64] Kristiansson M, Soop M, Saraste L, Sundqvist KG. Cytokines in stored red blood cell concentrates: promoters of systemic inflammation and simulators of acute transfusion reactions? *Acta Anaesthesiol Scand* 1996;40(4):496-501.

[65] Muylle L. The role of cytokines in blood transfusion reactions. *Blood reviews* 1995;9(2):77-83.

[66] Collard KJ. Is there a causal relationship between the receipt of blood transfusions and the development of chronic lung disease of prematurity? *Medical hypotheses* 2006;66(2):355-64.

[67] Isbister JP, Soyer A. Incidence and causes of hyperbilirubinaemia in a hospital population: with particular reference to blood transfusion. *The Medical journal of Australia* 1982;1(6):261-4.

[68] Isbister JP. Changes in laboratory parameters following transfusion of stored autologous blood. *Personal observations presented at the International Society of Blood Transfusion*, Sydney 1986 1986.

[69] Escobar GA, Cheng AM, Moore EE, et al. Stored Packed Red Blood Cell Transfusion Up-regulates Inflammatory Gene Expression in Circulating Leukocytes. *Annals of surgery* 2007;246(1):129-34.

[70] Ciesla DJ, Moore EE, Johnson JL, et al. Decreased progression of postinjury lung dysfunction to the acute respiratory distress syndrome and multiple organ failure. *Surgery* 2006;140(4):640-7; discussion 7-8.

[71] Smith HM, Farrow SJ, Ackerman JD, Stubbs JR, Sprung J. Cardiac arrests associated with hyperkalemia during red blood cell transfusion: a case series. *Anesthesia and analgesia* 2008;106(4):1062-9, table of contents.

[72] Aboudara MC, Hurst FP, Abbott KC, Perkins RM. Hyperkalemia After Packed Red Blood Cell Transfusion in Trauma Patients. *The Journal of trauma* 2008;64(2):S86-S91.

[73] Meikle A, Milne B. Management of prolonged QT interval during a massive transfusion: calcium, magnesium or both? *Canadian journal of anaesthesia = Journal canadien d'anesthesie* 2000;47(8):792-5.

[74] Nilsson KR, Berenholtz SM, Garrett-Mayer E, Dorman T, Klag MJ, Pronovost PJ. Association between venous thromboembolism and perioperative allogeneic transfusion. *Arch Surg* 2007;142(2):126-32; discussion 33.

[75] Twomley KM, Rao SV, Becker RC. Proinflammatory, immunomodulating, and prothrombotic properties of anemia and red blood cell transfusions. *Journal of thrombosis and thrombolysis* 2006;21(2):167-74.

[76] Grunenberg R, Kruger J. Analysis of cytokine profiles of stored CPDA-1 whole blood. *Infusionsther Transfusionsmed* 1995;22(5):292-4.

[77] Heddle NM. Pathophysiology of febrile nonhemolytic transfusion reactions. *Current opinion in hematology* 1999;6(6):420-6.

[78] Covin RB, Ambruso DR, England KM, et al. Hypotension and acute pulmonary insufficiency following transfusion of autologous red blood cells during surgery: a case report and review of the literature. *Transfusion medicine* (Oxford, England) 2004;14(5):375-83.

[79] Spiess BD. Risks of transfusion: outcome focus. *Transfusion* 2004;44(12 Suppl):4S-14S.

[80] Malone DL, Dunne J, Tracy JK, Putnam AT, Scalea TM, Napolitano LM. Blood transfusion, independent of shock severity, is associated with worse outcome in trauma. *The Journal of trauma* 2003;54(5):898-905; discussion -7.

[81] Goldman M, Webert KE, Arnold DM, Freedman J, Hannon J, Blajchman MA. Proceedings of a consensus conference: towards an understanding of TRALI. *Transfusion medicine reviews* 2005;19(1):2-31.

[82] Toy P, Lowell C. TRALI--definition, mechanisms, incidence and clinical relevance. *Best Pract Res Clin Anaesthesiol* 2007;21(2):183-93.

[83] Curtis BR, McFarland JG. Mechanisms of transfusion-related acute lung injury (TRALI): anti-leukocyte antibodies. *Critical care medicine* 2006;34(5 Suppl):S118-23.

[84] Bux J. Transfusion-related acute lung injury (TRALI): a serious adverse event of blood transfusion. *Vox sanguinis* 2005;89(1):1-10.

[85] Silliman CC, McLaughlin NJ. Transfusion-related acute lung injury. *Blood reviews* 2006;20(3):139-59.

[86] Silliman CC. The two-event model of transfusion-related acute lung injury. *Critical care medicine* 2006;34(5 Suppl):S124-31.

[87] Silliman CC, Kelher M. The role of endothelial activation in the pathogenesis of transfusion-related acute lung injury. *Transfusion* 2005;45(2 Suppl):109S-16S.

[88] Rael LT, Bar-Or R, Ambruso DR, et al. The effect of storage on the accumulation of oxidative biomarkers in donated packed red blood cells. *The Journal of trauma* 2009;66(1):76-81.

[89] Zilberberg MD, Carter C, Lefebvre P, et al. Red blood cell transfusions and the risk of ARDS among critically ill: a cohort study. *Crit Care* 2007;11(3):R63.

[90] Yilmaz M, Keegan MT, Iscimen R, et al. Toward the prevention of acute lung injury: Protocol-guided limitation of large tidal volume ventilation and inappropriate transfusion. *Critical care medicine* 2007;35(7):1660-6.

[91] Cherry T, Steciuk M, Reddy VV, Marques MB. Transfusion-related acute lung injury: past, present, and future. *American journal of clinical pathology* 2008;129(2):287-97.

[92] Triulzi DJ. Transfusion-related acute lung injury: current concepts for the clinician. *Anesthesia and analgesia* 2009;108(3):770-6.

[93] Spiess BD. Red Cell Transfusions and Guidelines: A Work in Progress. *Hematol Oncol Clin North Am* 2007;21(1):185-200.

[94] Practice guidelines for perioperative blood transfusion and adjuvant therapies: an updated report by the American Society of Anesthesiologists Task Force on Perioperative Blood Transfusion and Adjuvant Therapies. *Anesthesiology* 2006;105(1):198-208.

[95] Rao SV, Jollis JG, Harrington RA, et al. Relationship of blood transfusion and clinical outcomes in patients with acute coronary syndromes. *Jama* 2004;292(13):1555-62.
[96] Huber-Wagner S, Qvick M, Mussack T, et al. Massive blood transfusion and outcome in 1062 polytrauma patients: a prospective study based on the Trauma Registry of the German Trauma Society. *Vox sanguinis* 2007;92(1):69-78.
[97] Wettstein R, Erni D, Intaglietta M, Tsai AG. Rapid restoration of microcirculatory blood flow with hyperviscous and hyperoncotic solutions lowers the transfusion trigger in resuscitation from hemorrhagic shock. *Shock* (Augusta, Ga 2006;25(6):641-6.
[98] Cabrales P, Martini J, Intaglietta M, Tsai AG. Blood Viscosity Maintains Microvascular Conditions During Normovolemic Anemia Independent of Blood Oxygen Carrying Capacity. *American journal of physiology* 2006.
[99] Tsai AG, Cabrales P, Intaglietta M. Blood viscosity: a factor in tissue survival? *Critical care medicine* 2005;33(7):1662-3.
[100] Cabrales P, Tsai AG, Winslow RM, Intaglietta M. Extreme hemodilution with PEG-hemoglobin vs. PEG-albumin. *American journal of physiology* 2005;289(6):H2392-400.
[101] Cabrales P, Intaglietta M, Tsai AG. Increase plasma viscosity sustains microcirculation after resuscitation from hemorrhagic shock and continuous bleeding. *Shock* (Augusta, Ga 2005;23(6):549-55.
[102] Cabrales P, Martini J, Intaglietta M, Tsai AG. Blood viscosity maintains microvascular conditions during normovolemic anemia independent of blood oxygen-carrying capacity. *American journal of physiology* 2006;291(2):H581-90.
[103] Wettstein R, Tsai AG, Erni D, Lukyanov AN, Torchilin VP, Intaglietta M. Improving microcirculation is more effective than substitution of red blood cells to correct metabolic disorder in experimental hemorrhagic shock. *Shock* (Augusta, Ga 2004;21(3):235-40.
[104] Thyes C, Spahn DR. Current status of artificial O2 carriers. *Anesthesiol Clin North America* 2005;23(2):373-89, viii.
[105] Winslow RM. Targeted O2 delivery by low-p50 hemoglobin: a new basis for hemoglobin-based oxygen carriers. *Artificial cells, blood substitutes, and immobilization biotechnology* 2005;33(1):1-12.
[106] Wettstein R, Cabrales P, Erni D, Tsai AG, Winslow RM, Intaglietta M. Resuscitation from hemorrhagic shock with MalPEG-albumin: comparison with MalPEG-hemoglobin. *Shock* (Augusta, Ga 2004;22(4):351-7.
[107] Tsai AG, Cabrales P, Intaglietta M. Oxygen-carrying blood substitutes: a microvascular perspective. *Expert opinion on biological therapy* 2004;4(7):1147-57.
[108] Van Meter KW. A systematic review of the application of hyperbaric oxygen in the treatment of severe anemia: an evidence-based approach. *Undersea Hyperb Med* 2005;32(1):61-83.
[109] Meier J, Kemming GI, Kisch-Wedel H, Blum J, Pape A, Habler OP. Hyperoxic ventilation reduces six-hour mortality after partial fluid resuscitation from hemorrhagic shock. *Shock* (Augusta, Ga 2004;22(3):240-7.
[110] Bose D, Tejwani NC. Evolving trends in the care of polytrauma patients. *Injury* 2006;37(1):20-8.
[111] Nathens AB. Massive transfusion as a risk factor for acute lung injury: association or causation? *Critical care medicine* 2006;34(5 Suppl):S144-50.

[112] Moore FA, Moore EE, Sauaia A. Blood transfusion. An independent risk factor for postinjury multiple organ failure. *Arch Surg* 1997;132(6):620-4; discussion 4-5.
[113] Charles A, Shaikh AA, Walters M, Huehl S, Pomerantz R. Blood transfusion is an independent predictor of mortality after blunt trauma. *The American surgeon* 2007;73(1):1-5.
[114] Robinson WP, 3rd, Ahn J, Stiffler A, et al. Blood transfusion is an independent predictor of increased mortality in nonoperatively managed blunt hepatic and splenic injuries. *The Journal of trauma* 2005;58(3):437-45.
[115] Despotis GJ, Zhang L, Lublin DM. Transfusion Risks and Transfusion-related Pro-inflammatory Responses. *Hematol Oncol Clin North Am* 2007;21(1):147-61.
[116] Dunne JR, Malone DL, Tracy JK, Napolitano LM. Allogenic Blood Transfusion in the First 24 Hours after Trauma Is Associated with Increased Systemic Inflammatory Response Syndrome (SIRS) and Death. *Surgical infections* 2004;5(4):395-404.
[117] Friedlander MH, Simon R, Machiedo GW. The relationship of packed cell transfusion to red blood cell deformability in systemic inflammatory response syndrome patients. *Shock* (Augusta, Ga 1998;9(2):84-8.
[118] Weiskopf RB, Feiner J, Hopf H, et al. Fresh blood and aged stored blood are equally efficacious in immediately reversing anemia-induced brain oxygenation deficits in humans. *Anesthesiology* 2006;104(5):911-20.
[119] Raat NJ, Berends F, Verhoeven AJ, de Korte D, Ince C. The age of stored red blood cell concentrates at the time of transfusion. *Transfusion medicine* (Oxford, England) 2005;15(5):419-23.
[120] Gonzalez AM, Yazici I, Kusza K, Siemionow M. Effects of fresh versus banked blood transfusions on microcirculatory hemodynamics and tissue oxygenation in the rat cremaster model. *Surgery* 2007;141(5):630-9.
[121] Leal-Noval SR, Munoz-Gomez M, Arellano-Orden V, et al. Impact of age of transfused blood on cerebral oxygenation in male patients with severe traumatic brain injury. *Critical care medicine* 2008;36(4):1290-6.
[122] Marik PE, Sibbald WJ. Effect of stored-blood transfusion on oxygen delivery in patients with sepsis. *Jama* 1993;269(23):3024-9.
[123] Leal-Noval SR, Jara-Lopez I, Garcia-Garmendia JL, et al. Influence of erythrocyte concentrate storage time on postsurgical morbidity in cardiac surgery patients. *Anesthesiology* 2003;98(4):815-22.
[124] Raat NJ, Verhoeven AJ, Mik EG, et al. The effect of storage time of human red cells on intestinal microcirculatory oxygenation in a rat isovolemic exchange model. *Critical care medicine* 2005;33(1):39-45; discussion 238-9.
[125] Dzik W. Fresh blood for everyone? Balancing availability and quality of stored RBCs. *Transfusion medicine* (Oxford, England) 2008;18(4):260-5.
[126] Koch CG, Li L, Sessler DI, et al. Duration of red-cell storage and complications after cardiac surgery. *The New England journal of medicine* 2008;358(12):1229-39.
[127] Weinberg JA, McGwin G, Jr., Marques MB, et al. Transfusions in the less severely injured: does age of transfused blood affect outcomes? *The Journal of trauma* 2008;65(4):794-8.
[128] Upile T, Jerjes W, Sandison A, et al. The direct effects of stored blood products may worsen prognosis of cancer patients; shall we transfuse or not? An explanation of the adverse oncological consequences of blood product transfusion with a testable

hypothesis driven experimental research protocol. *Medical hypotheses* 2008;71(4):489-92.

[129] Atzil S, Arad M, Glasner A, et al. Blood transfusion promotes cancer progression: a critical role for aged erythrocytes. *Anesthesiology* 2008;109(6):989-97.

[130] Spahn DR, Holger M, Hofmann A, Isbister J. Patient Blood Management: The Pragmatic Solution for the Problems with Blood Transfusions. *Anesthesiolgy* 2008;109(6):951-3.

[131] Cauwenberghs S, van Pampus E, Curvers J, Akkerman JW, Heemskerk JW. Hemostatic and signaling functions of transfused platelets. *Transfusion medicine reviews* 2007;21(4):287-94.

[132] Isbister JP. Decision making in perioperative transfusion. *Transfus Apheresis Sci* 2002;27(1):19-28.

[133] Madjdpour C, Heindl V, Spahn DR. Risks, benefits, alternatives and indications of allogenic blood transfusions. *Minerva anestesiologica* 2006;72(5):283-98.

[134] Spahn DR. Strategies for transfusion therapy. *Best Pract Res Clin Anaesthesiol* 2004;18(4):661-73.

[135] Picker SM, Sturner SS, Oustianskaja L, Gathof BS. Leucodepletion leads to component-like storage stability of whole blood--suggesting its homologous use? *Vox sanguinis* 2004;87(3):173-81.

[136] Bratosin D, Leszczynski S, Sartiaux C, et al. Improved storage of erythrocytes by prior leukodepletion: flow cytometric evaluation of stored erythrocytes. *Cytometry* 2001;46(6):351-6.

[137] Wagner SJ, Myrup AC. Prestorage leucoreduction improves several in vitro red cell storage parameters following gamma irradiation. *Transfusion medicine* (Oxford, England) 2006;16(4):261-5.

[138] Frake PC, Smith HE, Chen LF, Biffl WL. Prestorage leukoreduction prevents accumulation of matrix metalloproteinase 9 in stored blood. *Arch Surg* 2006;141(4):396-400; discussion

[139] Gyongyossy-Issa MI, Weiss SL, Sowemimo-Coker SO, Garcez RB, Devine DV. Prestorage leukoreduction and low-temperature filtration reduce hemolysis of stored red cell concentrates. *Transfusion* 2005;45(1):90-6.

[140] Bessos H, Seghatchian J. Red cell storage lesion: the potential impact of storage-induced CD47 decline on immunomodulation and the survival of leucofiltered red cells. *Transfus Apheresis Sci* 2005;32(2):227-32.

[141] Obara S, Iwama H. Prestorage leukocyte reduction prevents the formation of microaggregates that occlude artificial capillary vessels. *Journal of critical care* 2004;19(3):179-86.

[142] Luk CS, Gray-Statchuk LA, Cepinkas G, Chin-Yee IH. WBC reduction reduces storage-associated RBC adhesion to human vascular endothelial cells under conditions of continuous flow in vitro. *Transfusion* 2003;43(2):151-6.

[143] Friese RS, Sperry JL, Phelan HA, Gentilello LM. The use of leukoreduced red blood cell products is associated with fewer infectious complications in trauma patients. *American journal of surgery* 2008;196(1):56-61.

[144] van de Watering L. What has universal leucodepletion given us: evidence from clinical trials? *Vox sanguinis* 2004;87 Suppl 2:139-42.

[145] Rosario MD, Rumsey EW, Arakaki G, Tanoue RE, McDanal J, McNamara JJ. Blood microaggregates and ultrafilters. *The Journal of trauma* 1978;18(7):498-506.

[146] James OF. The occurence and significance of microaggregates in stored blood. *European journal of intensive care medicine* 1976;2(4):163-6.

[147] Girdano J, Zinner M, Hobson RW, Gervin A. The effect of microaggregates in stored blood on canine pulmonary vascular resistance. *Surgery* 1976;80(5):617-23.

[148] Wilson K, Wilson M, Hebert PC, Graham I. The application of the precautionary principle to the blood system: the Canadian blood system's vCJD donor deferral policy. *Transfusion medicine reviews* 2003;17(2):89-94.

[149] Seghatchian J. nvCJD and leucodepletion: an overview. *Transfusion science* 2000;22(1-2):47-8.

In: Transfusion - Think About It
Editor: Trevor J. Cobain
ISBN 978-1-61668-969-8

Chapter 6

COAGULATION LESIONS IN WHOLE BLOOD AND COMPONENTS

James Thom and John Lown
Royal Perth Hospital, Perth, Western Australia.

ABSTRACT

Fresh unrefrigerated whole blood has been used successfully in situations of massive blood loss. It may have a greater haemostatic capacity than blood components and this has been examined by assessing the state of platelet activation and plasma coagulation parameters in fresh whole blood compared to other blood products. Platelet activation was measured using surface P-selectin expression by flow cytometry, the quantitation of platelet derived microvesicles, platelet dense granule staining and plasma levels of soluble CD40 ligand and soluble P-selectin. Platelet function was examined by optical aggregometry and plasma coagulation function was tested using the INR, aPTT, fibrinogen and D-dimer level. The activation state of platelets between products was significantly different. The platelets from fresh whole blood had lower surface P-selectin expression than those from red cell concentrates ($p = <0.0001$) and platelet concentrates ($p = <0.0001$). Soluble CD40L was significantly lower in fresh whole blood compared to platelet concentrates ($p = <0.0001$). There were no statistically significant differences in any of the coagulation parameters. Platelets from red cell concentrates and platelet concentrates are activated during production. The low level of activation of platelets in fresh unrefrigerated whole blood may contribute to the clinical efficacy observed in situations of massive transfusion.

INTRODUCTION

Increasingly non-human derived, therapeutic agents are becoming available to treat a range of acquired and congenital haemostatic abnormalities. These include recombinant coagulation proteins (aFVII, FVIII and FIX), DDAVP, vitamin K and aprotinin. However a range of blood components is still used routinely to prevent or arrest blood loss. Most commonly fresh frozen plasma (FFP) is used to replace factors depleted because of liver disease, warfarin therapy or blood loss. Red cell concentrates are given to correct bleeding associated with anaemia arising from various clinical, surgical and trauma settings. Cryoprecipitate can be used in von Willebrand's disorder to replace fibrinogen and platelet concentrates are used in thrombocytopenic patients.

In cases of massive blood loss, a coagulopathy may develop which can be difficult to control. The pathogenesis of this is multifactorial, being due to a mixture of vascular damage, consumption of coagulation proteins and loss of platelets. For a recent review see Levy 2006 [1]. These situations are generally managed by giving concentrated red cells to replace the oxygen carrying capacity and FFP, platelet concentrates and other products as appropriate to maintain haemostasis. An alternative approach to this may sometimes be the use of fresh whole blood.

The clinical value of fresh whole blood (ie unrefrigerated and less than 24 hours post collection) for uncontrolled haemorrhage has previously been reported [2]. Several other groups have noted improved haemostasis with fresh whole blood transfusions over red cell concentrates and other blood components [3-6].

It is possible that improved clinical efficacy is at least partly due to the superior function of platelets. As far back as 1985 Rodgers et al [7] found better platelet function in whole blood compared to whole blood derived platelet concentrates. Truilzi et al [8] demonstrated that the preparation of concentrates led to activation of platelets and expression of surface P-selectin, and that this activation was inversely proportional to platelet count increment one hour post transfusion. Holme et al [9] studied platelet activation in whole blood and in platelet concentrates prepared by apheresis. They found a ten fold higher level of surface P-selectin expression on platelets from concentrates but little in whole blood or platelet rich plasma prepared from whole blood by centrifugation. With isotopic survival studies they demonstrated this to be a predictor of platelet viability. However using surface P-selectin expression as well as platelet dense granule staining and enumeration of microvesicles, Wang et al [10] found platelets in concentrates to be activated immediately after preparation and Curvers et al [11] related this activation to decreased platelet responsiveness to physiological agonists.

As well as activation of platelets other factors may contribute to the efficacy of fresh whole blood as a therapeutic agent. Large procoagulant platelets can be lost in the preparation of platelet concentrate [4] and since it is recognised that platelets must be stored at room temperature to maintain their viability, blood should be fresh and unrefrigerated to maximise the therapeutic effect [12].

To examine these factors we compared platelet activation, platelet function and plasma coagulation parameters in unrefrigerated fresh whole blood (fresh WB), in refrigerated whole blood (refrigerated WB), in red cell concentrates (RCC) and in whole blood derived platelet concentrates (platelet concentrates).

PRODUCTS

Whole blood bags (n = 20) were processed at two time points. On the first occasion testing was performed as soon as the blood was received (fresh WB) which was a mean of 16 hrs 55 min post collection. The bags were then refrigerated overnight and retested as refrigerated WB after a mean of 17 hrs 30 min refrigeration, a mean total time of 34 hrs 25 min after collection. On each occasion the bag was well mixed by inversion and a sub sample of 30 mls was collected and the bag resealed. A full blood count, surface P-selectin expression on platelets and quantitation of platelet derived microvesicles (PDM) were performed on whole blood. Platelet rich plasma was prepared by centrifugation at 800g for 5 mins. The supernatant was removed and the blood re-centrifuged at 2000g for 10 minutes for platelet poor plasma. Platelet rich plasma was adjusted to a count of 250 x 10^9/l with platelet poor plasma prior to aggregometry testing. Platelet poor plasma was used to measure coagulation parameters. Aliquots were snap frozen and stored at –80°C for assay of soluble CD 40 ligand (sCD40L) and soluble P-selectin

Platelet concentrates (n = 20) were prepared by double centrifugation of donor whole blood donations at 22°C. The initial centrifugation was 1000g for 4.2 min and the second for 6 min at 2500g (Beckman J6 centrifuge, Beckman Coulter, Barcelona, Spain). Platelet concentrates were processed at one time point a mean of 24 hr 28 mins after collection. Platelet rich plasma was prepared as above and used for aggregometry, surface P-selectin expression and quantitation of PDM. Platelet poor plasma was used to measure coagulation parameters. Aliquots were snap frozen and stored at –80°C for assay of sCD40L and soluble P-selectin

RCC (n = 20) were prepared by a single centrifugation of whole blood at 2500g for 10 min in a Beckman J6 centrifuge (Beckman Coulter). They were tested for platelet surface P-selectin expression and PDM concentration a mean of 18 hr and 40 min post collection.

LABORATORY ANALYSES

Platelets were examined by flow cytometry in three ways:

a) Activated platelets were determined using FITC conjugated anti-glycoprotein IIIa (Becton Dickinson, Franklin Lakes, NJ, USA) as a platelet marker and PE conjugated anti CD62 (Becton Dickinson) to detect the activation marker surface P-selectin.
b) Platelet dense granule content was determined by labelling of platelets with mepacrine as previously described [13].
c) PDM were quantitated using FITC conjugated anti-glycoprotein IIIa (Becton Dickinson) as a platelet marker and gating on particles less than 1μm. Flow-Chek Fluorospheres (Beckman Coulter, Miami, USA) were added as an internal standard to allow quantitation.

All flow cytometry was performed on the Coulter EPICS XL-MCL flow cytometer (Beckman Coulter).

sCD40L and soluble P-selectin were measured in duplicate using commercially available ELISA assays (Bender MedSystems, Vienna, Austria).

Optical platelet aggregometry was performed using platelet rich plasma on the Chronolog 680 PICA aggregometer (Philadelphia, USA). Agonists, at the final concentration in the aggregometer cuvette, were 7μmol /L adrenaline, 4 μmol/L ADP, 1μg/ml collagen and 1mmol/L arachidonic acid. For the purposes of interpretation, an amplitude of 70% or greater was considered to be normal, 40 – 69% was designated slightly impaired and less than 40% markedly impaired.

Prothrombin time, aPTT, fibrinogen and D-dimers were assayed using standard procedures on the STA-R automated coagulation analyser (Diagnostica Stago, Asnières, France). Full blood counts were performed on the Cell Dyn Haematology analyser (Abbott Laboratories, IL, USA). Statistical analysis was performed using means, standard deviation and two tailed, equal variance Student's t-test. A p-value of ≤ 0.05 was considered significant.

PLATELET ACTIVATION

Markers of platelet activation, surface P-selectin expression and PDM, were significantly lower in fresh whole blood compared to RCC and platelet concentrates. After refrigeration there was a significant fall in PDM compared to fresh WB. Mepacrine staining of the platelet dense granules was significantly lower in platelet concentrates than in fresh WB. The results are detailed in table 1.

Table 1. Surface platelet activation markers in fresh WB, refrigerated WB, platelet concentrates and RCC. Mean (SD). P values are for comparisons with fresh WB.

	Surface P-selectin (%)	PDM × 10^8/l	Dense granule staining (%)
fresh WB	5.2 (3.7)	56.8 (27.3)	82.2 (5.8)
refrigerated WB	6.9 (4.7) not significant	38.0 (18.4) p = 0.0008	81.0(7.1) not significant
platelet concentrates	15.4 (6.7) p = <0.0001	854.48 (760.5) p = <0.0001	78.6 (8.2) p = 0.01
RCC	23.6 (10.5) p = <0.0001	244 (240.4) p = 0.0006	Not tested

Table 2. Soluble platelet activation markers in fresh WB, refrigerated WB and platelet concentrates. Mean (SD). P values are for comparisons with fresh WB.

	Soluble CD40L (ng/ml)	Soluble p-selectin (ng/ml)
fresh WB	2.1 (1.73)	287.7 (270.0)
refrigerated WB	2.2 (1.83) not significant	270.5 (235.7) not significant
platelet concentrates	10.4 (4.55) p = <0.0001	457.2 (347.7) not significant

PDM were also significantly higher in platelet concentrates than in RCC ($p = 0.001$) and surface P-selectin significantly lower ($p = 0.005$).

sCD40L was lower in fresh WB than in platelet concentrates (table 2). Soluble P-selectin in refrigerated WB was significantly lower than in platelet concentrates ($p = 0.04$).

Levels of sCD40L and soluble P-selectin were significantly correlated ($r = 0.346$, $p = 0.005$). There was no significant correlation between levels of sCD40L or soluble P-selectin with time post collection.

Platelet Aggregation

Platelet aggregation was profoundly reduced in all products. ADP aggregation (4 µmol/L) was markedly impaired in 82.6% of fresh WB, 91.3% of refrigerated WB and 100% of platelet concentrates ($p = 0.02$ fresh WB vs platelet concentrates). Adrenaline (7 µmol/L) induced aggregation was markedly impaired in 91.3% of fresh WB, 91.3% of refrigerated WB and 95% of platelet concentrates (not significant) and collagen (1 mg/L) markedly impaired in 86.9%, 95.7% and 95% (not significant) respectively. Platelets were more responsive to arachidonic acid (1mmol/L) however, with normal responses in 43.6% of fresh WB, 69.6% of refrigerated WB and 50% of platelet concentrates (not significant). The aggregation responses are shown in Figure 1. Platelet aggregation was not tested in RCC due to difficulty separating platelet rich plasma.

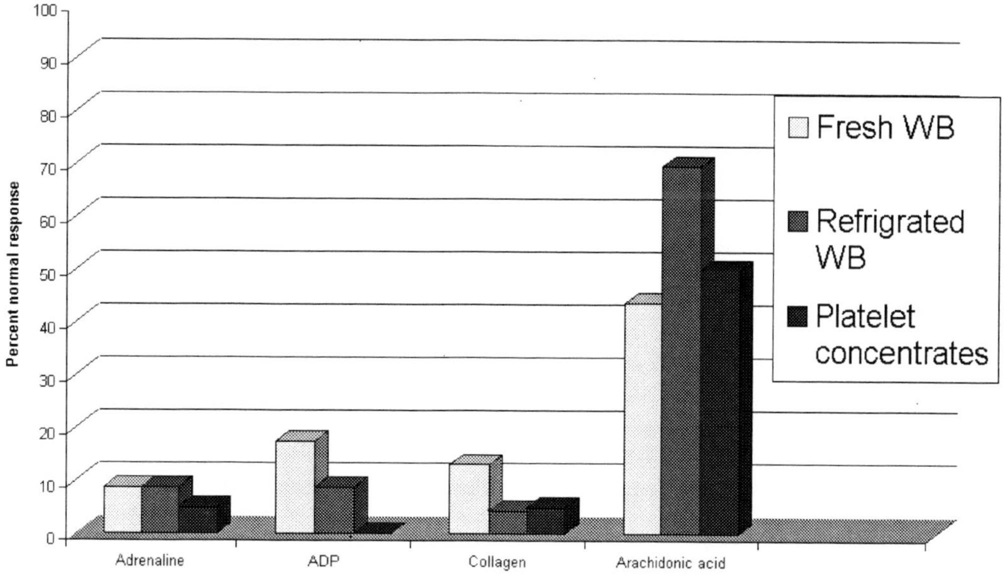

Figure 1. Percentage of normal response for platelet aggregation in fresh WB, refrigerated WB and platelet concentrates with Adrenaline (7µmol/L), ADP (4µmol/L), collagen (1mg/ml) and arachidonic acid (1mmol/L).

Coagulation Proteins

All measured coagulation parameters in fresh WB, refrigerated WB and platelet concentrates were within the normal ranges with no comparative statistically significant differences. There was no significant difference in the platelet count of fresh WB and refrigerated WB. The results are shown in Table 3.

Table 3. Coagulation parameters and platelet counts in whole blood and platelet concentrates. Mean (SD)

	INR	APTT(s)	D-Dimer mg/l	Fibrinogen g/l	Platelets x 10^9/L
Normal Range	**0.9 – 1.3**	**29.5 – 40.5**	**<0.4**	**2.0 – 4.1**	**150 – 400**
fresh WB	1.0 (0.09)	33.5 (3.0)	0.26 (0.10)	2.80 (0.4)	226 (50.3)
refrigerated WB	1.1 (0.08)	34.7 (3.6)	0.29 (0.1)	2.85 (0.4)	225 (49.5)
platelet concentrates	1.2 (0.1)	34.0 (4.7)	0.29 (0.5)	2.91(0.7)	Not tested

Discussion

In this study we compared platelet activation, platelet aggregation and plasma coagulation status in fresh WB, refrigerated WB, RCC and platelet concentrates. Processes involving centrifugation and separation of whole blood (RCC and platelet concentrates) significantly increased *in vitro* markers of platelet activation when compared to unmanipulated blood (fresh WB and refrigerated WB). This finding may in part provide an explanation for the occasional observed clinical efficacy of whole blood in situations of massive haemorrhage.

Whole blood is not usually the appropriate product for red blood cell or coagulation factor replacement. Blood donations are generally channeled into components to allow for specific therapies and extended storage. The production of multiple blood components from one donation is often the most efficient use of a scarce resource.

However it is important to use the most appropriate blood product for every situation. Fresh WB can be a complete product for the restoration of oxygen carrying and haemostatic capacity. It has been successfully used to control massive life threatening bleeds [2] as well as in elective situations where massive transfusion is expected [3,4]. When multiple blood components are required, often in a large number, fresh WB blood may also have a logistic advantage.

Our results suggest that the preparation of fresh WB is virtually free of any processes that would lead to the activation of platelets. Whereas centrifugation, which is necessary to prepare both RCC and platelet concentrates, is a relatively traumatic procedure which may reduce platelet viability [8,11]. It may also be that large platelets, lost in the preparation of platelet concentrates and which are present in fresh WB, enhance its haemostatic ability [5].

Cellular Markers of Activation

Differences between the products were pronounced when markers of platelet activation were examined. The alpha granule membrane marker P-selectin was significantly increased in RCC and platelet concentrates compared to fresh WB and was higher in RCC than in platelet concentrates. This *in vitro* study did not assess the haemostatic potential, or half life of the infused products. Previously it has been shown that platelets expressing P-selectin are rapidly removed from circulation. Triulzi et al [8] found transfused activated platelets to be less effective in increasing platelet count *in vivo* and Culvers et al [11] showed activated platelets have reduced aggregation.

Mepacrine staining of dense granules was significantly decreased in platelet concentrates when compared to fresh WB suggesting degranulation during the preparation of platelets.

The concentration of PDM was increased approximately 5 fold in RCC and 15 fold in platelet concentrates compared to fresh WB, most likely caused by the shear stress of centrifugation necessary for production. The effect of transfusion of products rich in PDM is unknown. Microvesicles have been reported to be both procoagulant and anticoagulant [14] and have been implicated in the development of atherosclerosis [15]. It is likely that PDM generated by mechanical forces are different to those circulating in disease states. Xiao et al found that PDM produced by thrombin treatment of platelets increased platelet aggregability when added to washed platelets but PDM produced by freeze/thawing did not [16]. In a recent study PDM isolated from patients undergoing cardiac surgery were highly thrombogenic whereas PDM from normal individuals were not [17]. Transfusion of PDM in platelet concentrates is of uncertain clinical value. Procoagulant PDM have been demonstrated to improve *in vitro* platelet aggregation [16] and to encourage venous thrombus formation in rats [17] but it may be that they have a short half life *in vivo* being rapidly removed from circulation by P-selectin adhesion to monocytes [18].

Plasma Markers of Activation

Soluble P-selectin and sCD40L are blood markers of platelet activation. On stimulation granular P-selectin is initially expressed on the platelet surface then rapidly shed [19]. Similarly CD40 ligand is translocated to the platelet surface on activation then more slowly cleaved and released as sCD40L. [20]. In our study there was a highly significant increase in sCD40L in platelet concentrates with a smaller increase in soluble P-selectin compared to fresh WB and refrigerated WB. There was no significant correlation between the age of the products and the levels of the soluble activation markers suggesting that activation occurred during the preparation of the platelet concentrates.

Platelet Aggregation

Platelet aggregation was profoundly disturbed in all preparations with minimal response to adrenaline, ADP and collagen. This decrease in activity was most likely an aging effect due to the time elapsed prior to testing. The aggregation of platelets by these agonists is a multi step process dependent on both membrane receptors and internal signaling pathways for the production of thromboxane A_2. Arachidonic acid however is more directly converted into thromboxane A_2 and approximately half of the products retained a normal response to this agonist which was not significantly different between the groups.

One of the limitations of fresh whole blood is the short shelf life of 24 hours after which refrigeration is necessary to extend shelf life but this has been shown to reduce platelet function [12]. In this study overnight refrigeration of fresh WB led to a significant reduction in PDM and an observed, but not significant, increase in surface P-selectin expression. There was an observed increase in arachidonic acid induced aggregation after refrigeration although this was not statistically significant. There was no significant difference in the level of sCD40L or soluble P-selectin after refrigeration. However platelet activation in refrigerated WB was still substantially less than RCC or platelet concentrates. It may be of value to further evaluate the use of refrigerated whole blood.

Plasma Coagulation Proteins

Plasma coagulation parameters were all within normal ranges with no significant differences in plasma from fresh WB, refrigerated WB and platelet concentrates. Therefore it is unlikely that plasma factors play a major role in the efficacy of the different products.

Study Limitations

This was a relatively small in vitro study. One of the parameters used to assess the activation of platelets surface P-selectin expression has until recently been considered the gold standard marker of platelet activation. However activated platelets may lose their surface P-selectin over time [21] or adhere to white blood cells via P-selectin glycoprotein ligand-1 [19]. The formation of platelet-leucocyte aggregates, particularly platelet-monocytes complexes, has been reported to be a more reliable marker of activation [21] and should be used in future studies.

Conclusion

Platelets from either RCC or platelet concentrates express higher levels of surface P-selectin, have higher circulating levels of shed activation markers and have much higher levels of PDM relative to fresh WB. Platelets in fresh WB are closer to the normal physiological state and this may account for the reduced rate of haemorrhage that has been observed when fresh WB is used in cases of massive transfusion. Given the fact that multiple components can not be produced from a whole blood donation beyond 24 hours, when viewed from a Blood Donor Service perspective, it is essential that the clinical circumstances for using non-refrigerated whole blood are well defined. Carefully designed randomised studies should further inform the appropriate use of fresh WB.

REFERENCES

[1] Levy, J H. Massive transfusion coagulopathy. *Semin Hematol,* 2006 43 (suppl 1), s59 – s63.

[2] Erber, WN; Tan, J; Grey, D; Lown, JA. Use of unrefrigerated fresh whole blood in massive transfusion. *Med J Aust,* 1996 165, 11-13.

[3] Lavee, J; Martinowitz, U; Mohr, R; Goor, DA; Golan, M; Langsam, J; Malik, Z; Savion, N. The effect of transfusion of fresh whole blood versus platelet concentrates after cardiac operations. A scanning electron microscope study of platelet aggregation on extracellular matrix. *J Thorac Cardiovasc Surg,* 1989 97, 204-212.

[4] Manno, CS; Hedberg, KW; Kim, HC; Bunin, GR; Nicolson, N; Jobes, D; Schwartz, E; Norwood, WI. Comparison of the hemostatic effects of fresh whole blood, stored whole blood, and components after open heart surgery in children. *Blood,* 1991 77, 930-936.

[5] Mohr, R; Goor, DA; Yellin, A; Moshkovitz,Y; Shinfeld, A; Martinowitz, U. Fresh blood units contain large potent platelets that improve hemostasis after open heart operations. *Ann Thorac Surg,* 1992 53, 650-654.

[6] Erber, WN. Massive blood transfusion in the elective surgical setting. *Transfusion and Apheresis Science*, 2002 27, 83 – 92.

[7] Rodgers, SE; Lloyd, JV; Russell, WJ. Platelet function in platelet concentrates and in whole blood. *Anaesth Intens Care*, 1985 13, 355-361.

[8] Triulzi, DJ; Kickler, TS; Braine, HG. Detection and significance of alpha granule membrane protein 140 expression on platelets collected by apheresis. *Transfusion*, 1992 32, 529 – 533.

[9] Holme, S; Sweeney, JD; Sawyer, S; Elfath, MD. The expression of p-selectin during collection, processing and storage of platelet concentrates: relationship to loss of in vivo viability. *Transfusion,* 1997 37, 12 – 17.

[10] Wang, C; Mody, M; Herst, R; Sher, G; Freedman, J. Flow cytometric analysis of platelet function in stored platelet concentrates. *Transfus Sci*, 1999 20, 129 – 139.

[11] Curvers, J; van Pampus, ECM; Feijge, MAH; Rombout-Sestrienkova, E; Giesen, PLA; Heemskerk, JWM. Decreased responsiveness and development of activation markers of PLTs stored in plasma. *Transfusion*, 2004 44, 49 – 58.

[12] Golan, M; Modan, M; Lavee, J; Martinowitz, U; Savion, N; Goor, DA; Mohr, R. Transfusion of fresh whole blood stored (4 degrees C) for short period fails to improve platelet aggregation on extracellular matrix and clinical haemostasis after cardiopulmonary bypass. *J Thorac Cardiovasc Surg*, 1990 99, 354-360.

[13] Gordon, N; Thom, J; Cole, C; Baker R. Rapid detection of hereditary and acquired platelet storage pool deficiency by flow cytometry. *Brit J Haematol*, 1995 89,117-123.

[14]Tans, G; Rosing, J; Thomassen, MC; Heeb, MJ; Zwaal, RFA; Griffin, JH. Comparison of anticoagulant and procoagulant activities of stimulated platelets and platelet derived microvesicles. *Blood*, 1991 77, 2641–2648.

[15]Nomura, S; Tandon, NN; Nakamura, T; Cone, J; Fukuhara, S; Kambayashi, J. High-shear-stress-induced activation of platelets and microparticles enhances expression of cell adhesion molecules in THP-1 and endothelial cells. *Atherosclerosis*, 2001 158, 277–287.

[16]Xiao, H; Jepkorir, CJ; Harvey, K; Remick, DG. Thrombin-induced platelet microparticles improved the aggregability of cryopreserved platelets. *Cryobiology*, 2002 44, 179–188.

[17]Biró, É; Sturk-Maquelin, K N; Vogel, GMT; Meuleman, DG; Smit, M J; Hack, CE; Sturk, A; Nieuwland, R. Human cell-derived microparticles promote thrombus formation *in vivo* in a tissue factor-dependent manner. *J Thromb Haemost*, 2003 1, 2561 – 2568.

[18]McEver, RP. P-selectin/PSGL-1 and other interactions between platelets, leucocytes and endothelium.:In Michelson A D, Ed. *Platelets*. San Diego: Academic Press; 2002, 139 – 155.

[19]André, P. P-selectin in haemostasis. *Brit J Haematol*, 2004 126, 298 – 306.

[20]Prasad, KS; Andre, P; Yan,Y; Phillips, DR. The platelet CD40L/GP IIb-IIIa axis in atherothrombotic disease. *Curr Opin Hematol*, 2003 10, 356 – 361.

[21]Michelson, A; Barnard, M; Krueger, LA; Valeri, C; Furman, M. Circulating monocyte-platelet aggregates are a more sensitive marker of in vivo platelet activation than platelet surface P-selectin: Studies in baboons, human coronary intervention and human acute myocardial infarction. *Circulation*, 2001 104, 1533-1537.

In: Transfusion - Think About It
Editor: Trevor J. Cobain
ISBN 978-1-61668-969-8

Chapter 7

NON-REFRIGERATED FULLY TESTED WHOLE BLOOD – AN OPTION IN THE INITIAL DEBRIDEMENT OF MAJOR BURNS?

B. Carnley
Royal Perth Hospital, Perth, Western Australia.

ABSTRACT

The planning and delivery of blood and blood products during episodes of massive transfusion remains as a challenging scenario, that may need to be considered in the setting of a disaster response plan. In this setting, an argument can be made in the support of the delivery of fully tested non-refrigerated whole blood as an alternative to traditional blood component therapy. The following chapter outlines these arguments. The use of fully tested non-refrigerated whole blood, including production planning, delivery and haematological effectiveness of the product, as part of a disaster response plan implemented following the Bali bomb explosions of 2002, is presented to illustrate the use of the product.

INTRODUCTION

Clinical and transfusion staff aim to deliver the most appropriate blood product to patients, tailored to the clinical circumstances faced by the individual.

The motivation to achieve this aim is powered by issues relating to blood product supply and the need to ensure that blood, as a scarce resource, is utilised in the most efficient manner. Fractionation of whole blood into a number of components is a recognised element of efficient blood product utilisation. Component therapy facilitates the efficient use of donated whole blood in situations where the clinical need is restricted to an isolated or limited range of deficiencies. An example of this process working efficiently relates to the treatment of isolated anaemia; such patients are given red cell concentrates, and the plasma from the donated whole blood unit is "saved" to correct coagulation factor deficits in another individual or fractionated to produce other products. The provision of red cells, platelets and plasma as individual components is an approach that aims to supply the greatest number of individuals with components derived from a small donor population. Component therapy aims to address problems that relate to blood and blood product supply and assumes that one donor provides products to a number of recipients.

The need to safely supply an absolute number of components is generally recognised as the major priority of transfusion services. In contrast, consumer demand issues relating to the exact type of product requested by treating clinicians (eg single donor versus pooled platelets and product age), have traditionally been viewed at a lower priority when compared with the issues relating to efficient inventory management and the supply of a safe blood product.

Further more, the relative importance of criteria used to assess quality in a blood product differ between the organisations that provide blood and blood products and the clinicians that request those products. From a supply perspective a quality product is a safe product. For instance, a quality product has the lowest risk of bacterial and viral infection transmission. From a demand perspective, the quality aspects of a blood product relate to the immediate clinical effect of the product. A quality blood product stops bleeding (by increasing platelet levels or clotting factor activity) or improves oxygenation (by increasing haemoglobin concentration).

While the advantages relating to efficient inventory management associated with component therapy are clear, it is possible to argue that component therapy may not be the optimum product for use in situations where there is the expectation of a massive transfusion event (>10 units of product transfused). These arguments relate both to supply and quality of the product.

Major burn debridement is a semi-elective procedure in which a massive transfusion is generally expected. This clinical scenario may be encountered following a major disaster and the consideration of the transfusion needs may be a part of a disaster management plan. Major burn debridement provides a clinical example of a situation that highlights the limitations of component therapy and illustrates the rationale for considering alternative to component therapy. The use of non refrigerated fully tested whole blood (NRFTWB aka Fresh Blood) described here in, demonstrates that an alternative to component blood product therapy is available and that it can be produced and delivered as part of a disaster response plan.

Transfusion Therapy and Haemostatic defects in Burns Debridement – A Predictable Problem

Situations of high surgical blood loss such as major burn (>20%TBSA) debridement are commonly associated with large transfusion requirements. Blood loss may be extremely rapid and the haemostatic defects multi-factorial in nature. In these settings the defects are rarely uni-dimensional, as the surgical team may be confronted by anaemia coexisting with thrombocytopaenia, hypofibrinogenaemia, and coagulation factor deficiency. In the authors' experience the infusion of 10 to 20 units of packed red cells, numerous units of platelets, fresh frozen plasma and cryoprecipitate are often required in order to provide adequate transfusion support to patients with major burns undergoing debridement. It is important to recognise that component therapy is being used to replace whole blood loss rather than an isolated deficiency of haemoglobin, platelets or clotting factors. In this situation, one individual may receive the red cell, platelet and plasma components derived from whole blood donated by many different donors.

The normal expectation of bleeding and coagulation disturbances in severely burnt patients undergoing burn debridement is in part outlined in the work of Niemi [1]. This group prospectively evaluated haemostasis of 13 severely burnt patients undergoing excision of burns and skin grafting. The blood products required, in relation to the number of packed cells transfused were assessed in conjunction with assessments of coagulation factor levels and platelet concentration. For every 4 units of packed red cells transfused beyond 8 units, increasing numbers of units of platelet concentrates and fresh frozen plasma were required. When 12 units of packed red cells were transfused, a mean of 5.5 units of fresh frozen plasma units and 4.9 units of platelet concentrates were also transfused. The haemostatic abnormalities were proportional to the amount of blood product delivered and included depression of levels of factors II, V, VII, VIII and X and fibrinogen. Platelet counts were significantly decreased after transfusion of 8 units of packed cells to a mean of 59 (range 28-110) $x10^9/L$.

Despite most burn debridement surgery occurring within 4 to 8 days of the injury as a semi-elective procedure and the associated expectation of a massive transfusion event (>10 unit transfusion), this situation remains a considerable challenge to clinicians and transfusion staff alike.

Logistic difficulties may be generated by the need to deliver large volumes of blood components. Problems may arise due to difficulties in handling multiple units of blood products, both in theatre and in the transfusion unit. In addition, the delivery of large volumes of different blood components exposes the recipient to multiple donors, increasing the risk of infection, antibody production and other complications of transfusion. These potential problems arise as a direct consequence of component therapy.

Disturbance of thermal regulation associated with the debridement of extensive burns necessitates the heating of burns theatre suites, to avoid hypothermia. In this setting, fluid warmers are used to elevate the temperature of refrigerated blood component products during the process of transfusion to reduce the problems of hypothermia and adding a further layer of logistical complexity to transfusion management.

In addition to the practical disadvantages in using component therapy in the management of massive blood loss, there are issues relating to the quality of components available for transfusion. Unless a special request for fresh products is made, it is standard practice at the Australian Red Cross Blood Service to issue units of blood product closest to expiry. The storage of blood components is associated with progressive deterioration in quality of product. The oxygen carrying capacity of red cells falls with increasing storage times. Platelet function falls in platelet donations with time [2]. While the policy of releasing product that is closest to expiration date, is an effective inventory management tool, it can be argued that the least effective components may be delivered to the patients that actually need the best quality product.

Given that the degree of blood loss and haemostatic defects associated with major burn debridement and the associated expectation of a massive transfusion event, there is a clear need to consider potential blood product requirements while planning the procedure with a view to ensuring the availability of the optimum blood product(s) to manage the situation.

THE ALTERNATIVE TO COMPONENT THERAPY

Whole blood is a potential alternative to individual component therapy in the management of massive transfusion. While reports of whole blood use in major burn debridement are lacking, there are reports of the use of this product in other settings. Whole blood reported as a treatment of coagulopathy in field surgical care [3] during military conflict, cardiac surgery [4] and liver transplantation surgery [5]. In liver transplantation surgery, a procedure that like burn debridement is also associated with high transfusion requirements, the use of whole blood has been associated with fewer donor exposures [5].

Previous empirical experience with ultrafresh whole blood [6], a product of last resort, has demonstrated the superiority and effectiveness of warm whole blood, when compared with use of individual refrigerated blood components. Ultrafresh whole blood has however been criticised due to the lack of donor and product infectious screening prior to transfusion.

Non refrigerated fully tested whole blood is an alternative product produced by the Australian Red Cross Blood Service (ARCBS) in Perth, Western Australia, that meets all infectious screening and manufacturing safety standards required by the Therapeutic Goods Administration. This product represents an alternative option to component therapy, for use in the transfusion support for patients undergoing major burn debridement. A product comparison of NRFTWB and ultrafresh whole blood is presented in Table 1.

At a practical level there are a number of potential theoretical advantages associated with the use of warm whole blood over component therapy in burn debridement surgery. These include the potential need to handle a reduced number of products in the transfusion laboratory and the theatre environment. There is no need to warm the product as it has not been refrigerated, removing the need for fluid warmers.

In addition to the potential practical advantages associated with use of whole blood, there is some evidence indicating that the quality of the platelets in a unit of whole blood is superior to that of a component product. These differences provide some scientific basis upon which to believe that whole blood may be better than component therapy.

Differences in platelet size in whole blood units compared with platelet concentrates may be important. Platelets in platelet concentrates prepared from whole blood collections are smaller and haemostatically less viable than the larger platelets which are trapped in the packed red cell component [7].

The differences may relate to the effect of centrifugation in platelet concentrate production. Fresh blood units, shown to contain large potent platelets have been documented to improve haemostasis after open heart operations [8]. In the setting of open heart surgery it has been shown that these fresh packed cells have better platelet function and result in less bleeding than platelet concentrates [4].

Fresh whole blood is a potential source of a significant number of platelets.

Lavee et al demonstrated that the transfusion of 1 unit of fresh whole blood is associated with an equivalent increase in platelet count when compared with the transfusion of 6 conventionally prepared platelet concentrates [7].

The platelet storage lesion is well recognised. Platelet concentrates stored at room temperature undergo shape change and metabolic changes as a function of storage time, collection and agitation method. These changes include disc to sphere change, diminished adhesion and aggregation responses and changes in metabolic factors such as loss of membrane lipids that reduce platelet function [9,10,11]. One advantage associated with the use of NRFTWB relates to the potential for the platelet fraction within the whole blood to be delivered at an earlier time post donation than the component product that is currently available, with associated reduced potential for storage defects.

Table 1. Comparison of Non Refrigerated Fully Tested Whole Blood and Ultrafresh whole blood

	Non refrigerated Fully Tested Whole Blood	Ultrafresh Whole blood
Producer	ARCBS and requires careful planning re donor identification, timing of collection and product processing	"Hospital In House" product of last resort donors identified at the time of need from theatre and laboratory staff and unit collected
Donor screening	Formal as per routine ARCBS screening	No formal screening
Donation testing	Nucleic acid testing for HBV,HCV and HIV completed on the product prior to release.	Donor specimens collected prior to donation and a sample of the transfused product are tested after release of the product
Storage	Room Temperature (20-24°C) for up to 24 hours then refrigerated	Transfused immediately, excess is refrigerated for up to 24 hours post donation
Irradiation	Possible	Not Possible
Shelf life	21 days	24 hours post donation

ARCBS - Australian Red Cross Blood Service.

Bali Terrorism and Transfusion Therapy

The Bali bomb explosions in October 2002 presented an unprecedented challenge for a number of Burns / Plastic Surgery Units across Australia. The management of a cohort of six patients aged 15 to 42 years with 25 – 85% TBSA burns admitted to Royal Perth Hospital, illustrates the use of NRFTWB in the management of expected massive transfusion events associated with major burn debridement as part of a disaster management plan.

Following notification of the event, a multi-disciplinary working group comprising Surgical, Anaesthetic, Intensive Care, Haematology, Hospital Transfusion service and

ARCBS staff was established to plan the surgical intervention. NRFTWB was selected as the optimal blood product for use during the surgery, based on previous experience with ultrafresh whole blood in the setting of massive transfusion [6] and the reasons outlined above. On a case by case basis, an estimate of expected intra-operative blood loss and transfusion requirements was made based on the previous use of component blood product support. The multi-disciplinary working group estimated that a total of 110 units of NRFTWB would be required for the surgery. Expected blood loss on a case by case basis is outlined in Table 2.

Table 2. Predicted Product Requirements during initial debridement surgery

% TBSA involved	Blood Group	Predicted number of units of NRFTWB required
85	O pos	20
83	B pos	20
60	O pos	20
60	A pos	20
60	AB pos	20
28	A pos	10

TBSA – Total Body Surface area burn;
NRFTWB- Non refrigerated fully tested whole blood.

In addition to the major burns and blast injury, all patients in this cohort had bilateral perforated tympanic membranes and multiple minor fragmentation wounds and abrasions. Additional injuries included a large buttock fragmentation wound, an open wrist laceration and a right leg compartment syndrome. All patients underwent complete debridement of their burn injuries in one surgical episode within seven days of the initial injuries as planned.

The ARCBS was able to facilitate the donation, microbiological screening and delivery of 138 units of whole blood over a four day period over which initial debridement surgery was performed. Whole Blood was collected from suitably accredited donors. Donors were allocated appointment times to allow for maximum use of the blood whilst enabling full production and testing of donated units. Apart from the blood that was required for the weekend it was usually possible to produce the fresh whole blood without excessive overtime staff payment.

Transfused blood followed all the requirements of the Code of Good Manufacturing Practice (cGMP) and Council of Europe Guidelines (2002) [12]. After collection, the whole blood was maintained at room temperature 20-24°C in a controlled temperature room used for platelet storage. All blood was either transfused within a period of 24 hours from collection (NRFTWB) or was stored at 2-6°C after this time (refrigerated whole blood (RWB). RWB was assigned a 21 day shelf life and was available for transfusion to hospital in and outpatients. All products were tested for the usual viral, and serological markers as for all other transfusible blood products in Australia.

In all cases, clinical observation of blood loss in association with interpretation of ancillary laboratory data by the anaesthetist during the intra-operative period, provided the basis of the decision to transfuse NRFTWB. The number of units of NRFTWB transfused to each patient compared with the percentage burns and duration of surgery is shown in Table 3. No other blood products were required intra-operatively, 2 units of fresh frozen plasma were transfused to 1 patient in the immediate pre-operative period. No units were transfused to any of the patients in the cohort in the first 12 hours post operation.

Table 3. Products used during the intra-operative period and duration of surgery

% TBSA involved	Blood Group	Predicted number of units of NRFTWB required	Number of units of NRFTWB transfused	Operation duration
85	O pos	20	17	10 ;15
83	B pos	20	13	6:30
60	O pos	20	13	8:00
60	A pos	20	10	5:35
60	AB pos	20	7	5:00
28	A pos	10	7	5:00

TBSA – Total Body Surface area; NRFTWB- Non refrigerated fully tested whole blood.

Based on the authors' previous experience with major burns, it would appear that the use of NRFTWB was associated with the use of smaller numbers of transfused products when compared with the use of component therapy. This is in keeping with the experience of whole blood transfusion in the setting of liver transplantation [5].

Given the lack of experience with NRFTWB, it is not unexpected that a greater number of units of whole blood were requested than transfused, as reflected by the crossmatched : transfused ratio (C:T) of 1.86, where the intended recipient was a member of the survey cohort. It is important to note that estimations of blood product use during the initial debridement surgery were based on the experience of members of the working group in using packed cells and other component therapy to replace blood loss. If faced by a similar set of circumstances again in the future it could be anticipated that fewer units of NRFTWB could be requested for use during debridement surgery. Despite this, the overall C:T ratio of 1.21 indicates that whole blood that was not used by the cohort was not wasted. This overall C:T ratio was considered to be acceptable given the unique and unpredictable nature of the circumstances that were confronted.

Laboratory monitoring, requested at the time of debridement surgery based on clinical utility as determined by anaesthetic staff, indicated that haemoglobin and platelet counts along with coagulation profiles remained at levels that may not have been expected if component transfusion therapy had been utilised.

Five of the 6 patients undergoing debridement ended their procedures with higher haemoglobins than at the commencement and one patient with 85% TBSA burns who was not anaemic pre-operatively had a haemoglobin of 87g/L postoperatively. The haemoglobin range during the intra-operative period was 77 to 132 g/L.

During the intra-operative period, 5 of 6 patients maintained a platelet count of greater than 50 with 4 of these greater than $100x10^9/L$ without transfusion of platelet concentrates. One patient was thrombocytopaenic ($22x10^9/l$) preoperatively and maintained an improving platelet count intra-operatively rising to 85 x 10^9 /L at the post-operative period whilst being transfused with 13 units of fresh whole blood.

All patients maintained a normal or near normal international normalised ratio during the intra-operative period (result range 1.2 to 1.4).

All patients maintained an essentially normal activated partial thromboplastin time intra-operatively (result range 29.4 – 40.9 seconds), one patient having a marginal elevation at 42 seconds postoperatively. No patients required haemostatic support other than fresh whole blood.

Whilst there was a statistically significant (p=0.05) fall in fibrinogen levels across the designated time periods (Table 4), all patients maintained levels of fibrinogen above the lower limit of the normal range throughout the pre, intra and post operative periods.

Table 4. Statistical analysis - difference of paired means

Result Pair	Paired Differences					Significance (2-tailed) p value
	Mean	S.D	Standard error of mean	95% CI of difference (lower)	95% CI of difference (upper)	
aPTT intra - post	0.008	4.457	1.818	-4.66	4.68	0.997
aPTT intra - pre	-0.725	3.00	1.225	-3.875	2.425	0.580
INR intra -post	-0.15	0.103	0.042	-0.123	0.093	0.735
INR intra-pre	-0.15	0.103	0.042	-0.123	0.093	0.735
Fibrinogen intra-post	1.760	0.867	0.354	0.85	2.67	**0.004**
Fibrinogen intra-pre	-2.407	0.937	0.383	-3.390	-1.424	**0.001**
Hb intra-post	-10.4	24.3	9.94	-35.97	15.13	0.343
Hb intra-pre	2.083	14.864	6.068	-13.52	17.682	0.745
Plt intra - pre	2.27	28.304	11.56	-27.44	31.97	0.852
Plt intra - post	2.27	28.304	11.56	-27.44	31.97	0.852

aPTT-Activated Partial Thromboplastin Time; INR-International Normalised Ratio; Hb-Haemoglobin g/L; Plt-platelet count x10^9 / L; Pre-preoperative period; Intra-intraoperative period; Post-post operative.

SURVIVAL DATA

Two patients died from overwhelming sepsis at day 4 and day 56 post initial debridement surgery. The extent of the burns in these two cases was 85% and 83% TBSA respectively.

Striking and non Quantifiable Aspects of NRFTWB use

The situation described necessitated the implementation of a disaster plan which identified the need for additional staffing in the transfusion and coagulation units to cover the expected increase in demand for blood product and laboratory testing results. Additional resources included two scientists allocated to the transfusion and coagulation laboratories, and a dedicated patient care assistant to facilitate delivery of blood products to the theatre suite and intensive care units. Extra staff were not required, as an expected spike in workload did not eventuate during the period of the initial debridement surgery. Anaesthetic staff commented on the convenience due to reduced product handling associated with the use of NRFTWB. Intensive care staff noted that patients appeared more stable than expected on arrival into the unit following debridement. The surgical staff noted a striking difference during the surgery, with reduced blood loss and the absence of increasing oozing that traditionally develops intra-operatively in association with conventional transfusion therapy. Haemostasis was reported by surgical staff to be considerably better than they had expected. Application and adherence of the split skin grafts appeared to be improved in association with the observation of reduced blood ooze from the debrided wound bed.

Barriers to the Wide Spread Use of Non-Refrigerated Fully Tested Whole Blood

Evidence Gap and the Lack of Case Controlled Randomised Studies

The situation described here was a first for Royal Perth Hospital and includes a set of circumstances that has made identification of a relevant historical control group extremely difficult if not impossible. The cases described included major burns and trauma, and were cases that were denied comprehensive medical care for a period of approximately 24 hours prior to reaching a major teaching hospital. This type of delay is exceptional in the context of current burns management. Comparison of product use in the treatment of other patients injured in the described event and treated at other sites throughout Australia, was limited due to differences in surgical techniques.

A randomised study of component therapy in comparison with whole blood transfusion in the setting of burn debridement has to date, not been undertaken. Accordingly, unequivocal, scientifically rigorous proof of reduced donor exposure and stability of haematological profiling related to the use of NRFTWB is not available. The use of NRFTWB in the cohort described does however provide a basis on which to consider further study of this blood product.

Limitations of Whole Blood

Enthusiasm for the use of NRFTWB is tempered by the recognition that use is limited by the need to identify donors and plan donation times in relation to the proposed time of delivery of the released product. In Western Australia the shortest donation to delivery time for blood products is approximately eight hours. Accordingly, the use of non-refrigerated whole blood is currently restricted to elective surgery in which massive blood loss is expected. Stocks of non-refrigerated whole blood are not available at short notice for transfusion in the setting of acute trauma management.

There has been anecdotal evidence that citrate toxicity has decreased in multiple transfusion with the utilisation of packed red cells. Citrate toxicity whilst not recognised in this cohort remains a possibility that must be considered in massive transfusion involving whole blood.

Issues relating to blood group become particularly important when transfusing red cells that include plasma. One of the patients above was blood group AB. On most occasions this patient could have been transfused with group A red cells. The large volume of plasma, containing Anti-B in group A whole blood necessitated the transfusion of group AB whole blood. This has obvious implications on donor availability and inventory management.

Finally, there are potential cost implications relating to the provision of NRFTWB. In order to have whole blood available for semi – elective surgery there may be a requirement to have donors arrive at the collection centre, be interviewed, bled, tested, blood processed and issued, and cross matched at times that may be outside usual working hours. This has the potential to add substantial costs to production.

Conclusion

Whole Blood remains a transfusion option in the setting of semi-elective surgery that is associated with an expectation of massive transfusion. In the authors experience the transfusion of NRFTWB in the setting of major burn debridement was associated with minimal disturbance to coagulation profiles, haemoglobin concentrations and platelet numbers. There may be advantages in terms of reduced donor exposure and efficient blood product use when this blood product is used in preference to component therapy in the setting of major burn debridement. In addition there was a perceived patient benefit recognised by the operating surgeons, anaesthetists and intensive care physicians in addition to recognition of the ease of the blood product handling and administration in the operating suite.

The impact of NRFTWB in the prevention of coagulopathy and the cost effectiveness of this therapy, clearly requires further study so as to confirm the role of NRFTWB as a cost effective, clinically efficacious therapy for use in the debridement of major burns.

References

[1] Niemi, T, Svartling, N, Syrjala, M, et al. Haemostatic disturbances in burned patients during the early excision and skin grafting. *Blood coagulation and Fibrinolysis* 1998, 9, 19-28.

[2] Shukla SD, Morrison WJ, Klachko DM. Response to platelet activating factor in human platelets stored and aged in plasma. *Transfusion* 1989;29:528 –533.

[3] O'Sullivan J. Trauma-induced coagulopathy and treatment in Kosovo. *Military Medicine* 2001: 166; 362-365.

[4] Laine E, Stedman R, Calhoun L et al. Comparison of RBC and FFP with whole blood during liver transplantation surgery. *Transfusion* 2003;43:322-327.
[5] Erber WN, Tan J, Grey D, et al. Use of unrefrigerated whole blood in massive transfusion. *Med J Australia* 1996; 165: 11 – 13.
[6] Mohr R, Martinowitz V, Lavee J, et al. The Haemostatic effect of transfusing fresh whole blood versus platelet concentrates after cardiac operations. *Journal of Thoracic and Cardiovascular Surgery*, 1988, 96, 530-534.
[7] Mohr R, Goor DA, Yellin A et al. Fresh blood units contain large platelets that improve haemostasis after open heart operations. *Annals of Thoracic Surgery*, 1992, 53, 650 – 654.
[8] Levee J, Martinowitz V, Mohr R, et al. The effect of transfusion of fresh whole blood versus platelet concentrations after cardiac operations. *Journal of Thoracic and Cardiovascular Surgery*, 1989, 97, 204-212.
[9] Bertolini F, Murphy S. A multicentre inspection of the swirling phenomenon in platelet concentrates prepared in routine practice: Biomedical excellence for safer transfusion (BEST) working party of the international Society for Blood Transfusion. *Transfusion* 1996;36:128 –32.
[10]Rosenfield BA, Herfel B, Faraday N et al. Effects of storage time on quantitative and qualitative platelet function in transfusion. *Anaesthesiology* 1995;83:1167 – 72.
[11]Koener TA, Cunningham MT, Zhong DS. The role of membrane lipid in the platelet storage lesion. *Blood Cells* 1992;18:481-97.
[12]Guide to the preparation, use and quality assurance of blood components. 8th edition, *Council of Europe Publishing*, January 2002.

ACKNOWLEDGMENTS

The generous assistance of the following individuals with respect to the preparation of the Manuscript is gratefully acknowledged:

Associate Professor Richard Herrmann, Mrs Sue Finch and Mr John Lown, Mrs Maurene Trent — Haematology Department, Royal Perth Hospital

Dr Trevor Cobain, Ms Sandra Boyd — Australian Red Cross Blood Service, Perth

Professor Fiona Wood and Ms Anna Goodwin – Walters — Burns Unit, Royal Perth Hospital

In: Transfusion - Think About It
Editor: Trevor J. Cobain
ISBN 978-1-61668-969-8

Chapter 8

APHERESIS AND WHOLE BLOOD DERIVED PLATELETS: WHICH PRODUCT IS BEST?

Nancy M. Heddle*[*] *and Katerina Pavenski
Department of Medicine McMaster University, Hamilton Ontario, Canada;
Canadian Blood Services and McMaster University, Hamilton Ontario, Canada.

ABSTRACT

There are two approaches to the preparation of platelets: apheresis collections and the separation of platelets from whole blood by using either the buffy coat technique or centrifugation from platelet rich plasma [1]. The debate over which method results in the best platelet product has continued for many years and there is still no consensus on this issue. The answer will also be dependent on the definition of 'best' and whether the perspective is that of the supplier or the hospital transfusion service. Those who favour apheresis platelet products indicate that they are superior for many reasons including: reduction in the number of donor exposures for transfused recipients; improved bacterial safety profile; on-line/in-processing leukocyte reduction; and operational efficiencies and cost savings as multiple transfusion doses can be obtained from a single donation, and less laboratory time is needed in the hospital for preparation. Similarly, those who advocate platelets derived from whole blood describe some of the benefits as: lesser cost; optimal utilization of the entire 'volunteer' whole blood donation; and the ease of adaptability for pediatric and neonatal platelet dosing. However, even those who favour whole blood derived platelets can not necessarily agree on whether one preparation method is superior to the other. Table 1 summarizes some of the benefits proposed for the three types of platelet products.

In this chapter, the current methods for platelet production will be reviewed and considerations for selection of the manufacturing method and product will be presented

[*] Correspondence concerning this article should be addressed to: Nancy M Heddle MSc., FCSMLS(D), HSC 3N43, McMaster University, 1200 Main Street West, Hamilton, ON L8N 3Z5. Phone: (905) 525-9140 Ext 22126; Fax: (905) 524-2983; Email: heddlen@mcmaster.ca.

under the headings of bacterial screening, laboratory and clinical evidence to support the concepts of product equivalency or superiority, cost, and other considerations such as the need for CMV negative products and HLA matching.

Table 1. Summary of the proposed advantages and disadvantages of platelets prepared by apheresis and from whole blood donations by the PRP and BC methods

PRODUCT	PROPOSED ADVANTAGES	PROPOSED DISADVANTAGES
Apheresis Platelets	Single donor exposure Bacterial testing easily performed Facilitates providing CMV negative product HLA matched product can be provided Facilitates product issuing for transfusion (no pooling required) Inventory documentation is facilitated (one product to enter/select) Less space required for storage	More costly to collect
Platelets Prepared from Buffy Coats (BC)	Optimal utilization of the whole blood donation Less platelet injury than the PRP method Pre-storage pooling facilitates product issuing for transfusion Inventory documentation is facilitated (one product to enter/select) Less space required for storage More plasma can be diverted for fractionation Less costly (compared with apheresis)	Multiple donor exposures Prevalence of bacterial contamination may be higher than apheresis because of the pool
Platelets Prepared from Platelet Rich Plasma (PRP)	Optimal utilization of the whole blood donation Less costly (compared to apheresis) Facilitates dosing for pediatric and neonatal transfusions	Multiple donor exposures Prevalence of bacterial contamination may be higher than apheresis once pooling is performed Increased operational complexity for the hospital (more products to enter into inventory, pooling etc)

PLATELET PRODUCTION - METHODS OF PREPARATION

Platelet concentrates may be prepared from individual whole blood donations or collected from a single donor by apheresis. There are two types of whole blood derived platelets: platelets from platelet-rich plasma (PRP); and platelets prepared from buffy coats (BC). The PRP method has been the standard procedure used in North American since the late 1960s for platelet component manufacturing [1]. However, this North American profile is changing as one of the Canadian blood suppliers (Canadian Blood Services) is in the process of switching their manufacturing process to the BC method [2,3]. In Europe, the BC method is widely used and has been used for almost two decades.

With the PRP method, whole blood is collected and stored at room temperature for up to 8 hours. First, it is centrifuged at low speed ("soft spin", 2200 x g) for 3-4 minutes to yield red blood cells (RBC) and platelet-rich plasma. The PRP is extracted (through a leukoreduction filter if pre-storage leukoreduction is desired), and then centrifuged at high speed ("hard spin", 4000 x g) for 5 minutes separating plasma from platelets. The platelet pellet (with approximately 60 ml of residual plasma) is left undisturbed for 1 hour allowing the platelets to deaggregate. The platelets are then resuspended by gentle kneading of the bag or by placing the bag on a platelet agitator [4]. The platelet product is stored at room temperature under continuous agitation. Prior to transfusion, 4-6 units of platelets are pooled by the hospital blood bank to make an adult dose. Without the leukoreduction step, the white blood cell (WBC) count in a PRP derived product is in the order of 10^8 [5]. When leukoreduction is performed the targeted residual leukocyte threshold is $< 10^6$ leukocytes/product; however, in most products the residual leukocyte counts are even 1 or 2 logs lower. The red blood cell contamination within the product is minimal (usually less than 0.4 ml of packed red cells/product) [5].

With the buffy coat (BC) method, whole blood is rapidly cooled to room temperature on cooling trays following donation, then can be stored at room temperature for up to 24 hours before processing. The whole blood is centrifuged at high speed to yield packed red cells, the buffy coat layer, and plasma. The packed red cells and the plasma are extracted leaving the buffy coat layer which contains platelets, white cells and some of the red cells and plasma. Four to six buffy coats are then pooled using a sterile docking device along with plasma from one of the donors. The pooled buffy coat is centrifuged at low speed to separate platelet rich plasma from the red cells and leukocytes. The PRP is extracted through a leukoreduction filter if pre-storage leukoreduction is required. In some countries additive solution is used instead of plasma when preparing the BC product. The use of an additive solution allows for larger volumes of plasma to be collected and sent for fractionation. Compared with the PRP process, the buffy coat method yields a product with a similar platelet content and approximately 10% fewer contaminating white blood cells. There are significant logistical advantages to the BC method over the PRP method as summarized in Table 1 [1]. Both methods are illustrated in Figure 1.

In the apheresis method, the platelet component is prepared from the blood of a single donor by apheresis. Donors are connected via a peripheral line to a blood cell separator that withdraws and fractionates their whole blood, removes platelets to a separate container, and then returns the remaining platelet-depleted blood to the donor [4]. The process usually takes 1-2 hours. In some apheresis systems, platelets are collected as PRP and do not require resuspension; whereas, other systems produce a concentrated platelet pellet that must be resuspended [4]. There are a number of apheresis instruments available. Haemonetics' Mobile Collection (Hemonetics Corp., Braintree MA) utilizes a disposable plastic centrifuge chamber from which a layer of platelet-enriched plasma is siphoned into a collection bag. Caridian's Spectra and Trima (Caridian BCT, Lakewood CO) as well as the Baxter CS-3000 (Baxter Corp, Round Lake IL) uses a spinning channel with two-stage plastic inlays to initially separate the RBC from the PRP and then remove plasma from the platelet product. Baxter's Amicus separates PRP and then hyperconcentrates platelets along the collection bag wall prior to plasma resuspension in a storage container. Fresenius's ComTec (Fresenius Kabi, Bad Homburg, Germany) uses centrifugation with an innovative separation chamber. Each instrument uses a different in-process leukoreduction method [1]. Apheresis-derived platelets usually contain 10^4-10^6 leukocytes/product (which is <1% of the leukocytes in a non-leukoreduced platelet concentrate pool), and contains less than 0.5 ml of contaminating RBC [4]. Apheresis products are stored in the same way as BC and PRP platelets: at room temperature and with continuous agitation.

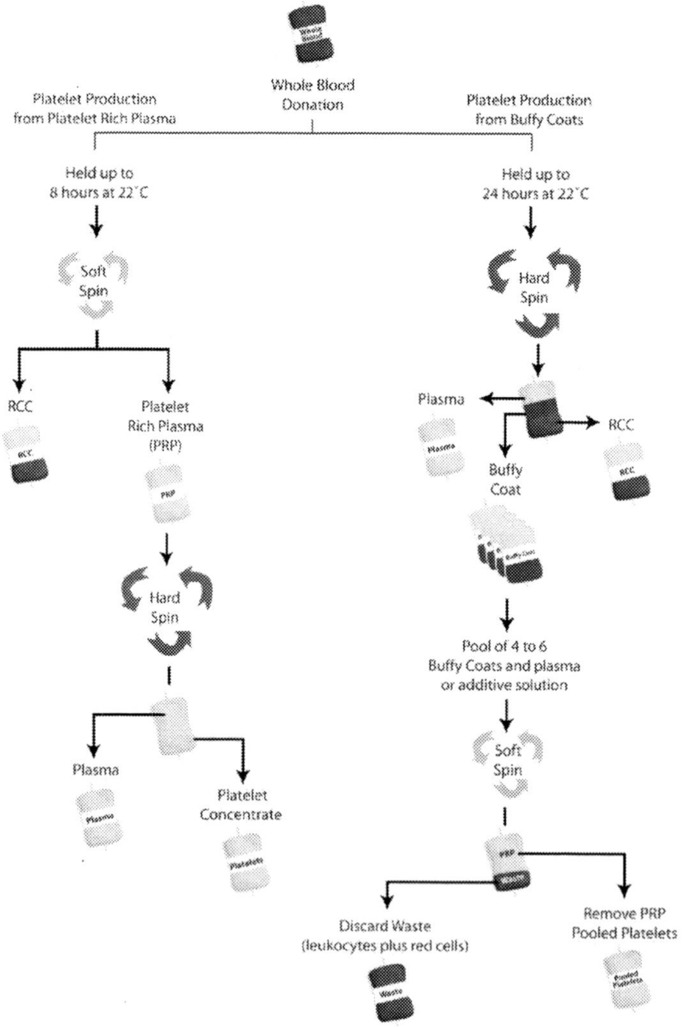

Figure 1. Illustration of the process for the preparation of platelets from whole blood using the platelet rich plasma method, and the buffy coat method.

All three methods yield a similar mean platelet concentration (approximately 1.5×10^9 platelets/ml). A single whole-blood derived platelet concentrate contains approximately $0.8\text{-}1.1 \times 10^{11}$ platelets [1], and has a volume of 45-65 ml [5]. The platelet concentration in a pooled product is approximately $3\text{-}6 \times 10^{11}$ cells [4]. Apheresis products contain $3\text{-}6 \times 10^{11}$ platelets and have a volume of 200 ml.; however, the apheresis technology also allows for collection of a high dose platelets (usually from donors with high normal platelet counts) product which can then be split yielding two therapeutic doses [1]. A pooled whole-blood derived product exposes a recipient to 4-6 donors while apheresis platelets only results in one donor exposure. Apheresis and BC derived platelets do not require in-hospital pooling and can be issued more rapidly. Apheresis and BC platelets may be associated with reduced wastage as these products are already pooled in a closed system compared to platelets prepared from PRP which have a shelf-life of only four hours after pooling. However, prestorage pooling of platelet prepared from PRP has been shown to be a safe and efficacious product and provides an option for dealing with the four hour shelf life.

BACTERIAL SCREENING OF PLATELETS

The prevalence of bacterial contamination in platelets is approximately 1 in 3,000 units transfused [6]. However, not all patients develop transfusion associated sepsis from these contaminated products. Available data suggests that transfusion associated bacterial sepsis occurs in approximately 1 in 25,000 platelet transfusions [6]. The risk of bacterial contamination also appears to be decreasing with the implementation of the diversion pouch which redirects the first few mls of blood at the start of collection into a satellite pouch preventing contamination of the entire unit of blood by a skin core contaminate; however, this technology can be applied to all methods of platelet collection [7]. Some studies have suggested that the prevalence of bacterial contamination is higher in whole-blood derived platelet concentrates than apheresis products [8,9]; however numerous other reports show variable results, some favouring a lower frequency with apheresis platelets, others favouring WBD platelets [4]. A recent report assessing bacterial contamination in over 52,000 platelet products demonstrated a similar frequency of confirmed positives in apheresis platelets and pooled platelet concentrates from whole blood (0.09% and 0.06% respectively) [10]. Regardless of the risk difference between products, bacterial contamination of platelets products is one of the more common causes of transfusion associated morbidity and mortality at the present time.

In 2003, the US was the first country to try and formally address this issue when the 22nd edition of the AABB Standards required that bacterial testing be performed on all platelets prior to release for transfusion [11]. Many countries throughout the world have also implemented a similar standard or are working towards this goal. To comply with such a standard is simplified with apheresis platelets and platelet prepared from buffy coats; however, bacterial testing of all platelets made from PRP has been challenging.

The most sensitive method currently applicable for routine bacterial detection in platelet products is bacterial culture. There are a number of automated culture systems commercially available to facilitate culture testing. One method detects bacterial growth by sensing CO_2 production (BacTec™ (BD, Franklin Lakes, NJ) and the other method relies on oxygen consumption to detect the micro-organisms (BacT/Alert®, bioMerieux Inc, Durham, NC) [12]. To be effective, sample volumes of 4-10 ml of product must be cultured. These culture methodologies are easily applied to apheresis platelets and whole blood derived platelets prepared by the BC method; however, bacterial testing of whole blood derived platelets from PRP is more challenging due to sampling, component management logistics, and cost [6]. One culture method that has been developed and is applicable to platelets prepared from PRP is the eBDS (Pall Corporation East Hills, NY) [13–15]. This system relies on the measurement of reduced oxygen levels in contaminated platelet components caused by microbial oxygen consumption during proliferation. The eBDS system does not require a large sample for testing and has been shown to have adequate sensitivity, good specificity and is a user-friendly system that is easy to perform [16]. However, many hospital transfusion services have opted for non-culture based methods that are less costly for testing platelets prepared from PRP. These methods include: staining techniques with microscopic examination (Gram, Wright or acridine orange) [17]; urine dipsticks (pH and glucose) [18]; and assessment of swirling. All of these methods have minimum detection thresholds that are at least 5-6 logs above the 10 colony-forming units/ml which is the threshold for the gold standard automated culture system; however, with the exception of swirling, they are all recognized as an acceptable approach for meeting current standards [19]. There are also non-culture based, commercially available methods that can be performed at the time that the platelet product is released for transfusion. The methodology of the Scansystem (Hemosystem, Marseille, France), involves direct detection of bacteria by labeling with a fluorescent dye and scanning with laser-based, solid-phase cytometry [20-22].

The feasibility of using a pool and store approach for whole blood derived platelets from PRP has also been investigated as pooled storage of this product would facilitate bacterial testing. *In vitro* measures of platelet function for PRP platelets that were pooled and stored for five days suggested no detrimental impact on platelet viability and function [23-25]. More recently a randomized controlled trial has been performed looking at the impact of the PRP platelet pool and store technique on the 18 to 24 hour CCI in patients with chemotherapy induced thrombocytopenia [26]. The study was designed as a non-inferiority study and the results showed that the pool and store technique was not inferior to PRP platelets stored individually and pooled just prior to transfusion. Similar rates for bleeding and adverse events were also observed with the two types of product storage. There is currently a platelet bag licensed in the US for storing PRP platelets as a pool. The pool and store approach allows for more sensitive techniques for bacterial detection to be applied to the pooled PRP platelet product [1].

The challenges and costs associated with bacterial detection in platelet products are important consideration from both the blood supplier and hospital perspective when selecting the type of platelet product to make available for transfusion [17]. Future advances to reducing the risk of transfusing bacterially contaminated platelet products are inevitable and both apheresis and BC derived platelets lend themselves to experimental pathogen inactivation systems to decrease this risk [1,27].

In Vitro Comparisons of Platelet Products

Platelets viability diminishes with duration of storage. This is usually accompanied by changes in platelet morphology/activation state, metabolic capacity and physiologic responsiveness (referred to as the storage lesion). Development of the platelet storage lesion is thought to be related to the collection technique, storage conditions, and post-collection manipulation [4]. Several reports showed that leukocyte reduction procedures do not adversely affect platelet quality during storage [28,29]. In contrast, centrifugation during the manufacturing process, can expose platelets to shear stress conditions that result in the release of cytosolic LDH and stimulate platelet release reaction. Platelet granule release may be evidenced by elaboration of β-thromboglobulin into plasma or expression of P-selectin (CD62P) on the platelet membrane [4]. Because centrifugation is variable depending on the method of platelet preparation, numerous studies have been performed looking at a variety of *in vitro* markers that may indicate the quality of the stored platelet product.

There are numerous *in vitro* tests that have been used to compare the *in vitro* storage characteristics of platelet products prepared by different methods. These tests include: metabolic markers; assessment of shape change, platelet activation, and physiological markers [30,31]. Regardless of the tests performed, all three types of platelet concentrates have similar *in-vitro* characteristics by day five of storage [1]. However, this may not be true at the onset of storage. Studies have shown that PRP platelets have higher *in-vitro* markers of activation as evidenced by surface CD62P and CD63 expression, glycoprotein IIb/IIIa activation, loss of membrane glycoprotein Ib, and platelet factor 3 activity among others. Markers of activation are the lowest in BC platelets and intermediate in apheresis platelets. It has been suggested that the observation of less activation with BC platelets could be related to the first "soft spin" where platelets are centrifuged against a cushion of RBC instead of a plastic container. Activation in apheresis platelets may be related to the method used by the machines to harvest platelets [1]. There is one study showing that activated platelets produced persistently lower chromium labeled recoveries in normal volunteers [32]. However, no one has yet related the diverse effects of the processing and storage induced changes on aggregation and functional integrity to clinical outcomes in patients [33].

The major limitation of the *in vitro* studies to compare platelet product quality is the lack of a gold standard *in vitro* test that correlates well with *in vivo* effectiveness. At the present time maintenance of pH above a threshold of 6.0 has been shown to be the most critical factor that correlates with platelet viability [5]. One study suggests that at the end of storage, PRP platelets and apheresis platelets are more prone to develop a basic pH while BC platelets may become slightly acidic [34]; however, this observation was not confirmed in a recent study by Seghatchian et al [33]. Current *in vitro* test results suggest that there are few differences between platelet products prepared by apheresis and platelet products derived from whole blood (PRP and BC), and our interpretation of any differences observed is hindered by limited or no correlation of *in vitro* test results with clinical patient outcomes.

IN VIVO COMPARISON OF PLATELET PRODUCTS

The strongest evidence to compare the clinical effectiveness of different types of platelet products comes from randomized controlled trials (RCTs). There are a number of published RCTs that have compared apheresis platelets to whole blood derived platelets (PRP and/or BC), for the outcomes of: post transfusion corrected count increment; interval between transfusion; alloimmunization and refractoriness; and acute adverse reactions [35-45]. Recently a systematic review has been published summarizing these clinical trails and the evidence as to whether differences exist between the three types of products [46]. The findings with each of these outcomes are summarized below.

Post Transfusion Count Increment:

When the post transfusion increment is reported in clinical studies it is usually expressed as a corrected count increment (CCI). Calculation of the CCI is determined by dividing the increment (post-transfusion platelet count minus pre-transfusion platelet count x 10^9/L), by the total number of platelets in the platelet product and multiplying by the BSA. Hence, the CCI calculation accounts for the fact that patients have variable blood volumes and that the total number of platelets in the transfused product is not a standardized dose. Within 1 hour post-transfusion a CCI of $\geq$ 10 is considered acceptable and 18-24 hours post-transfusion the CCI should be $\geq$ 4.5 [47]. For the CCI measurement to be comparable and useful, it assumes that platelets can be accurately measured in the platelet product and BSA can be consistently determined. Recent reports suggest that variability exists when measuring platelets depending on the automated counter being used. Indeed in a study done by the BEST Collaborative (www.bestcollaborative.org), platelet counts performed in different laboratories on the same sample ranged from 808 x 10^9/L to 2219 x 10^9/L. Variation in estimating Body Surface Area (BSA) also occurs depending on the formula used. When BSA is calculated on a 6 foot 2 inch male weighing 180 pound using the various formulae on the website www.medal.org, the estimated BSA can range from 1.6 to 2.06 meters square. To illustrate the impact that the extreme values of BSA and product platelet count can have on the CCI, various calculations can be performed using an example post transfusion increment of 12 x 10^9/L. The CCI could be as low as 4.0 or as high as 14.0 when the different measurements are used.

In a single centre RCTs the variation around the CCI estimates are probably minimized as the type of counter and formula for BSA would be standardized; however, with multi-centre studies and inter-study comparisons, considerable variability could exist.

Recognizing this potential limitation, there were six RCTs that compared CCIs at 1- hour and/ or 18 – 24 hours post transfusion for apheresis and whole blood derived platelets [37,39,41-43,45]. The results of the mean CCIs by product type are summarized in Table2.

Table 2. Summary mean (SD) CCI at 1-hour and 18-24-hours in randomized controlled trials that compared different types of platelet products

Study	CCI 1-hour Mean (SD)			CCI 18- 24-hour Mean (SD)		
	WBD PRP	WBD BC	Apheresis	WBD PRP	WBD BC	Apheresis
Gmur (1983)	12.48 (3.70)		13.40 (4.80)	6.500 (2.90)		7.25 (4.00)
Anderson (1997)[+]	9.18 (16.22)	11.08 (16.34)	12.00 (14.64)	6.18 (23.80)	6.5 (22.75)	8.63 (21.51)
TRAP (1997)	12.2 (5.15)		14.70 (5.20)			
Kluter (1996)		15.87 (10.86)	18.48 (12.73)		11.86 (8.00)	10.78 (8.71)
Slichter (1998)	10.03 (5.93)		11.58 (8.12)			

[+] SD were calculated from SE and sample size reported in the paper.
WBD PRP = Whole blood derived platelets prepared from platelet rich plasma;
WBD BC = whole blood derived platelets prepared from buffy coats.

In all studies (n=4) where platelets from PRP were compared to apheresis platelets, the 1-hour and 18-24 hour CCIs were always higher with apheresis platelets. Higher 1-hour CCIs were also seen with apheresis platelets when compared to buffy coat platelets. PRP and BC platelets gave similar CCI results. Overall these results suggest that the CCI post transfusion (1 and 18-24 hours), is higher with apheresis platelets compared to whole blood derived platelets. This finding was also observed in two other RCTs investigating adverse events but reporting CCI as a secondary outcome [43,48]. In these studies the 18-24 hour CCI was reported as a dichotomous outcome where values $\geq$ 4.5 were considered successful and values below this threshold classified as unsuccessful. In both studies, the apheresis platelets had a success rate of approximately 53%; whereas, PRP platelets resulted in a successful CCI in only 35% of transfusions. To follow-up on this interesting observation, a radiolabelled survival and recovery study was performed in volunteers who donated autologous platelets by both apheresis and whole blood PRP techniques. The apheresis platelets had significantly better survival (32.9% better) and recovery (18.8% better) compared to platelets prepared from PRP [49]. These observations in volunteers and patients with leukemia, suggests that the apheresis platelet will results in a higher post transfusion platelet count. However, it is not known whether this observation translates into a longer interval between transfusions, fewer products being used, less bleeding, a shorter length of hospital stay, or has any long term impact on survival.

Alloimmunization and Refractoriness

These two terms are not independent as alloimmunization to HLA and/or platelet antigens can be associated with a poor post transfusion platelet increment (refractoriness); however, other clinical co-morbidities and treatment factors can also be responsible for refractoriness (i.e. fever, sepsis, DIC, bleeding, Amphotericin B administration; splenomegaly) [45,47,50]. There are three RCTs that have compared the effectiveness of apheresis versus whole blood derived platelets to prevent alloimmunization and/or refractoriness [36,37,41]. These studies were performed in patients receiving chemotherapy for acute leukemia. In the first study published in 1981 assessed the percentage of patients with alloimmunization following WBD PRP platelets and Apheresis platelet transfusions but did not assess refractoriness [36]. The second study from Germany (1983) compared apheresis platelets (non leukoreduced) to whole blood derived platelets prepared from platelet rich plasma [37]. The third study was a large multicentre study performed in the US where patients were randomized to one of four treatment arms. In three of the treatment arms whole blood platelets prepared from PRP were transfused: non leukoreduced; post-storage leukoreduced; and UVB treated platelets. The fourth treatment arm was post-storage leukoreduced apheresis platelets [41]. The proportions of patients with alloimmunization, refractoriness, and alloimmune-refractoriness by product type are summarized in Figure 2 a, b and c respectively.

The results from the study by Gmur et al [37] suggested that transfusion of apheresis platelets resulted in fewer patients with alloimmune refractoriness (14.8% for apheresis platelets versus 55.5% for platelets derived from PRP); however, the larger TRAP trial [41] reported similar percentages (4% for leukoreduced apheresis platelets and 3% for leukoreduced platelets derived from PRP). These currently available data suggests that rates of alloimmunization, refractoriness and alloimmune-refractoriness are similar with apheresis and PRP platelets. There are no data from buffy coat platelets looking at this outcome.

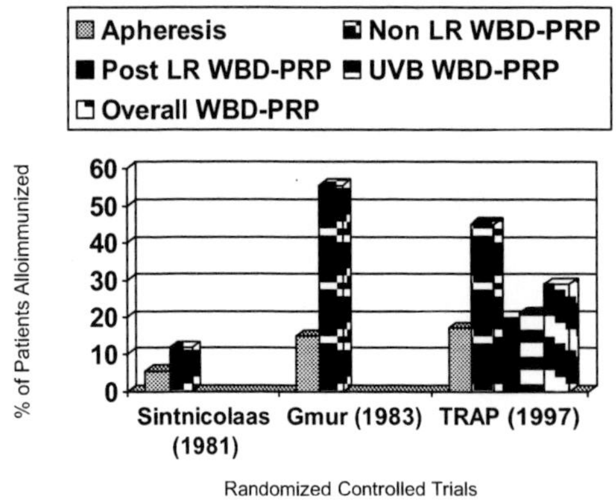

a

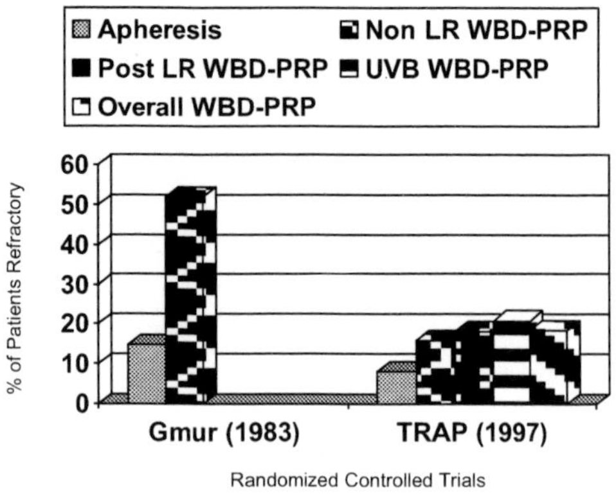

b

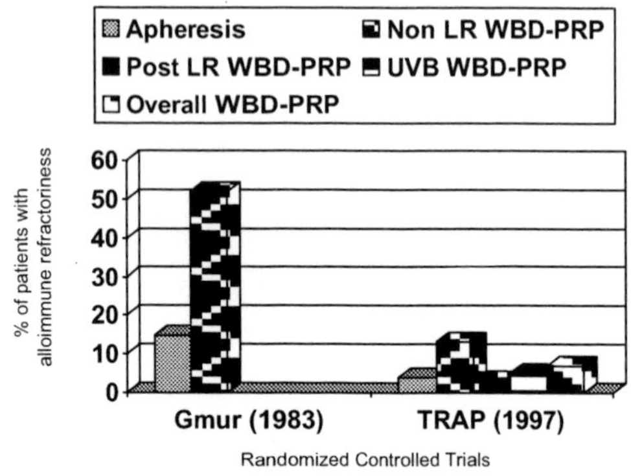

c

Figure 2. These figures represent the proportion of patients' who became alloimmunized (a), refractory (b), and developed alloimmune refractoriness (c) following the transfusion of various types of platelet products in randomized controlled trials assessing these outcomes. The total sample size of the studies were: Sintnicholaas (34 patients); Gmur (54 patients) and the TRAP study(530 patients). The blood products in the studies by Sintnicholaas and Gmur were non leukoreduced. The PRP platelets in the TRAP study were a mixture of non leukoreduced, post-storage leukoreduced and platelets treated with UVB light. The figures provide event frequencies for all the PRP platelets combined and for only the RPR platelets that were post-storage leukoreduced. The apheresis platelets were also post –storage leukoreduced; hence, the post-storage leukoreduced PRP platelets from TRAP provide a more appropriate comparison.

Acute Adverse Events

There are four clinical trials that provide information about the frequency of acute reactions following various types of platelet products [41-43]. Two other reports by Bishop [38] and Enright [44], provide additional information on the studies of Anderson and TRAP respectively. The methods of reporting in these trials are variable with some reports expressing the frequency of adverse event per patient, while others report reactions as a proportion of total transfusions. Figure 3 shows the frequency of acute adverse reactions per patient in the two studies reporting this outcome.

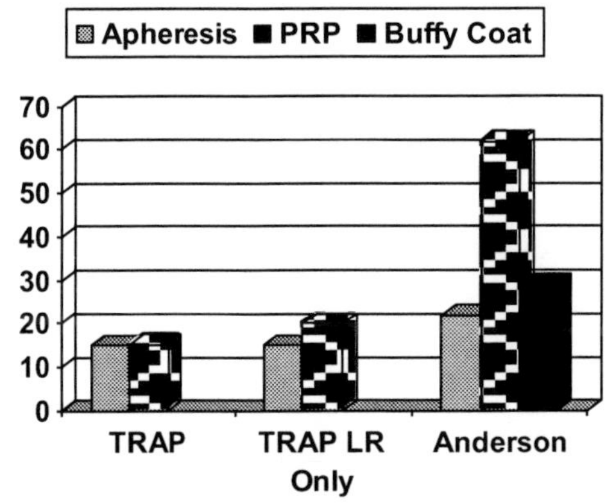

Figure 3. Bar graph indicating the frequency of acute adverse events per patient for the different platelet products.

The TRAP study results [41] are presented for all three arms using platelets from PRP and are also reported for only the post-storage leukoreduced products, providing a more valid comparison with the post-storage leukoreduced apheresis product. The results suggest that apheresis platelets may be associated with a lower frequency of reactions than platelets prepared from PRP. Only the study by Anderson [42] assessed reaction frequency to buffy coat platelets (29%) which was significantly lower than the frequency seen with platelets from PRP (62%). This is not surprising as the buffy coat methods of platelet preparation results in a 10% reduction in the number of leukocytes.

All four studies provide data on the frequency of reactions expressed as a percentage of platelet products transfused (Figure 4) [40-43].

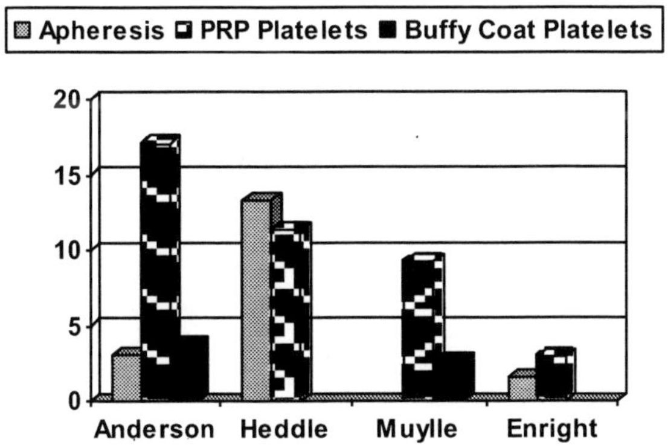

Figure 4. Bar graph indicating the frequency of adverse event per platelet transfusion for the different platelet products.

Reaction definitions used in these studies were variable: some investigators reported only severe events [41,42] while others reported all reactions (mild to severe) [43]. Some studies required a fever for a reaction to be documented as a febrile non-hemolytic transfusion reaction (FNHTR) [40-42]; whereas, one study reported FNHTR when symptoms developed regardless of a rise in temperature [43]. Although some studies showed that apheresis products had a lower reaction rate, interpretation of these data are difficult as product age and leukoreduction are factors know to influence the risk of an acute adverse events. The results suggest that buffy coat platelets have a lower frequency of reactions than PRP platelets when the products are not leukoreduced by filtration. The study by Heddle et al. [43] showed a similar reaction frequency with PRP and apheresis platelets when both products were pre-storage leukoreduced (11.4% and 13.3% respectively).

Other Outcomes

There have been no studies that have compared different types of platelet products for outcomes such as length of hospital stay, bleeding and mortality. Outcome studies using these endpoints would be useful for making evidence based decisions regarding the effectiveness of the different platelet types.

In summary, interpretation of existing data looking at clinical outcomes suggests that: 1) Buffy coat platelets are associated with fewer reactions than platelets prepared from PRP; 2) Apheresis platelets results in a higher 18-24 hour CCI than platelets prepared from whole blood; however, current data supporting this observation comes from one manufacturer's instrument; hence, generalizability of this finding to other instruments is unknown; and 3) There are no data to suggest differences in the frequency of alloimmunization and refractoriness based on the type of product transfused. Other outcomes that indicate long term impact and financial burdens are lacking, and current data only applies to patients with hematology malignancies and not other patient populations that required platelet transfusion support.

Cost

There are few published data about the cost of different types of platelet products, and costing that is available is often from the perspective of the blood supplier. In Canada, hospitals do not pay directly for blood products; however, the estimated costs for platelet products (± 10%)are apheresis platelets - $579; platelets from PRP - $112. The average cost of platelets in the US is slightly lower: $510/apheresis platelet and $64/PRP platelet [51]. There are no available costing data from hospital platelet transfusions that take into consideration adverse outcomes and the burden of such outcomes on hospital resources. Similarly, there is no information on the cost of platelet transfusions from the societal perspective taking into account donor related costs (travel, time off work, resources put into managing adverse events etc.).

Other Considerations

There are other circumstances where a particular method of platelet preparation may be preferable. Apheresis platelets are amenable to matching for HLA or HPA. They are also a product of choice for IgA deficient platelets, CMV negative platelets, and whenever reduced donor exposure is required. Apheresis platelets and BC platelets are suspended in a single donor's plasma; hence, adverse event resulting from a donor attribute could be more common or potentially more severe because of the large plasma volume. This theoretically could increases the risk of TRALI, or haemolysis related to transfusion of plasma with high titers of anti-A and/or anti-B. On the other hand, driven by concerns about TRALI, there has been a move in the UK and more recently in the US to use only male plasma for plasma products and platelets [52]. With the BC method, it would be possible to resuspend the platelets in plasma exclusively derived from male donors. With PRP method, this is not practical [3].

CONCLUSION

With so much work that has been accomplished to compare the efficacy and effectiveness of different platelet products, it is surprising and concerning that we still lack the knowledge to make evidence based decision as to the optimal platelet product or the equivalence of platelet products. There are some clinical data to suggest that one product is better than another for preventing adverse reactions, and improving post transfusion platelet count increments. However, we still lack data on the impact of these observations on the cost and demand for platelet products. Perhaps a more collaborative international approach for addressing these issues would provide evidence based solutions in a more timely manner.

ACKNOWLEDGMENT

The assistance of Laura Molnar, Diana Boye and Emmie Arnold during the preparation of this manuscript is acknowledged.

REFERENCES

[1] Vassallo RR, Murphy S. A critical comparison of platelet preparation methods. *Curr.Opin.Hematol.* 2006 Sep;13(5):323-30.
[2] Canadian Blood Services. Buffy Coat Production Method. In: *Canadian Blood Services [electronic mail system].* 2006 Dec.
[3] International Forum. Logistics of platelet concentrates. *Vox Sang.* 2007;92:160-81.
[4] Hillyer CD, et al. *Blood Banking and Transfusion Medicine: Basic Principles & Practice.* Churchill Livingstone; 2003.
[5] Mintz PD. *Transfusion Therapy: Clinical Principles and Practice.* AABB Press; 1999.
[6] Blajchman MA, Beckers EA, Dickmeiss E, Lin L, Moore G, Muylle L. Bacterial detection of platelets: current problems and possible resolutions. *Transfus.Med.Rev.* 2005 Oct;19(4):259-72.
[7] Transfusion Transmitted Injuries Section BSSaHCAIDCfIDPaCPHAoC. *Transfusion Transmitted Injuries Surveillance System: Program Report 2004-2005.* Her Majesty the Queen in Right of Canada, represented by the Minister of Health; 2008.

[8] Rebulla P. In vitro and in vivo properties of various types of platelets. *Vox Sang.* 1998;74 Suppl 2:217-22.
[9] Popovski MA. *Transfusion Reactions.* 2nd edition ed. AABB Press; 2001.1-468 p.
[10] Schrezenmeier H, et al. *Bacterial contamination of platelet concentrates: results of a prospective multicenter study comparing pooled whole blood-derived platelets and apheresis platelets* 2007 Feb 7.
[11] American Association of Blood Banks. *Standards for Blood Banks and Transfusion Services.* 22 ed. Bethesda; 2003.
[12] Riedel S, Siwek G, Beekmann SE, Richter SS, Raife T, Doern GV. Comparison of the BACTEC 9240 and BacT/Alert blood culture systems for detection of bacterial contamination in platelet concentrates. *J.Clin.Microbiol.* 2006 Jun;44(6):2262-4.
[13] Ortolano GA, Freundlich LF, Holme S, Russell RL, Cortus MA, Wilkins K, Nomura H, Chong C, Carmen R, Capetandes A, et al. Detection of bacteria in WBC-reduced PLT concentrates using percent oxygen as a marker for bacteria growth. *Transfusion* 2003 Sep;43(9):1276-85.
[14] Holme S, McAlister MB, Ortolano GA, Chong C, Cortus MA, Jacobs MR, Yomtovian R, Freundlich LF, Wenz B. Enhancement of a culture-based bacterial detection system (eBDS) for platelet products based on measurement of oxygen consumption. *Transfusion* 2005 Jun;45(6):984-93.
[15] McDonald CP, Pearce S, Wilkins K, Colvin J, Robbins S, Colley L, Taylor J, Barbara JA. Pall eBDS: an enhanced bacterial detection system for screening platelet concentrates. *Transfus.Med.* 2005 Aug;15(4):259-68.
[16] Schmidt M, Hourfar MK, Nicol SB, Wahl A, Heck J, Weis C, Tonn T, Spengler HP, Montag T, Seifried E, et al. A comparison of three rapid bacterial detection methods under simulated real-life conditions. *Transfusion* 2006 Aug;46(8):1367-73.
[17] Yomtovian R, Jacobs MR. Gram Stain and Culture Surveillance-Significant Findings and Clinical Implications. In: *Food and Drug Administration, Workshop on Bacterial Contamination of Platelets [electronic mail system].* 1999 Sep 24.
[18] Werch JB, Mhawech P, Stager CE, Banez EI, Lichtiger B. Detecting bacteria in platelet concentrates by use of reagent strips. *Transfusion* 2002 Aug;42(8):1027-31.
[19] Unknown. Detection of Bacterial Contamination in Platelet Components. *Blood Bulletin* 2003 Dec;6(4):1-2.
[20] Morel P, Deschaseaux M, Bertrand X, Naegelen C, Talon D. Detection of bacterial contamination in platelet concentrates using Scansytem: first results. *Transfusion 42[Suppl],* 40S. 2002. Ref Type: Abstract
[21] Ribault S, Harper K, Grave L, Lafontaine C, Nannini P, Raimondo A, Faure IB. Rapid screening method for detection of bacteria in platelet concentrates. *J.Clin.Microbiol.* 2004 May;42(5):1903-8.
[22] McDonald CP, Colvin J, Robbins S, Barbara JA. Use of a solid-phase fluorescent cytometric technique for the detection of bacteria in platelet concentrates. *Transfus.Med.* 2005 Jun;15(3):175-83.
[23] Snyder EL, Stack G, Napychank P, Roberts S. Storage of pooled platelet concentrates. In vitro and in vivo analysis. *Transfusion* 1989 Jun;29(5):390-5.
[24] Moroff G, Holme S, Dabay MH, Sawyer S, Heaton WA, Law P, Alsop P. Storage of pools of six and eight platelet concentrates. *Transfusion* 1993 May;33(5):374-8.

[25]Heddle NM, Barty RL, Sigouin CS, Boye DM, Nelson EJ, Blajchman MA, Kelton JG. In vitro evaluation of prestorage pooled leukoreduced whole blood-derived platelets stored for up to 7 days. *Transfusion* 2005 Jun;45(6):904-10.

[26]Heddle NM, Cook RJ, Blajchman MA, Barty RL, Sigouin CS, Boye DM, Nelson EJ, Kelton JG. Assessing the effectiveness of whole blood-derived platelets stored as a pool: a randomized block noninferiority trial. *Transfusion* 2005 Jun;45(6):896-903.

[27]Klein HG. Pathogen inactivation technology: cleansing the blood supply. *J.Intern.Med.* 2005 Mar;257(3):224-37.

[28]Sweeney JD, Holme S, Stromberg RR, Heaton WA. In vitro and in vivo effects of prestorage filtration of apheresis platelets. *Transfusion* 1995 Feb;35(2):125-30.

[29]Dumont LJ, AuBuchon JP, Whitley P, Herschel LH, Johnson A, McNeil D, Sawyer S, Roger JC. Seven-day storage of single-donor platelets: recovery and survival in an autologous transfusion study. *Transfusion* 2002 Jul;42(7):847-54.

[30]Murphy S, Rebulla P, Bertolini F, Holme S, Moroff G, Snyder E, Stromberg R. In vitro assessment of the quality of stored platelet concentrates. The BEST (Biomedical Excellence for Safer Transfusion) Task Force of the International Society of Blood Transfusion. *Transfus.Med.Rev.* 1994 Jan;8(1):29-36.

[31]Seghatchian J, Krailadsiri P. The platelet storage lesion. *Transfus.Med.Rev.* 1997 Apr;11(2):130-44.

[32]Rinder HM, Murphy M, Mitchell JG, Stocks J, Ault KA, Hillman RS. Progressive platelet activation with storage: evidence for shortened survival of activated platelets after transfusion. *Transfusion* 1991 Jun;31(5):409-14.

[33]Segatchian J. A new platelet storage lesion index based on paired samples, without and with EDTA and cell counting: comparison of three types of leukoreduced preparations. *Transfusion and Apheresis Science 35*, 283-292. 2006. Ref Type: Abstract.

[34]Vasconcelos E, Figueiredo AC, Seghatchian J. Quality of platelet concentrates derived by platelet rich plasma, buffy coat and Apheresis. *Transfus.Apher.Sci.* 2003 Aug;29(1):13-6.

[35]Kakaiya A. Alloimmunization following apheresis platelets vs pooled plt concentrates Transfusions: A prospective randomized study. *Transfusion*. 1981. Ref Type: Abstract.

[36]Sintnicolaas K, Vriesendorp HM, Sizoo W, Stenfert Kroese WF, Haije WG, Hop WC, Abels J, Lowenberg B. Delayed alloimmunisation by random single donor platelet transfusions. A randomised study to compare single donor and multiple donor platelet transfusions in cancer patients with severe thrombocytopenia. *Lancet* 1981 Apr 4;1(8223):750-4.

[37]Gmur J, von FA, Osterwalder B, Honegger H, Hormann A, Sauter C, Deubelbeiss K, Berchtold W, Metaxas M, Scali G, et al. Delayed alloimmunization using random single donor platelet transfusions: a prospective study in thrombocytopenic patients with acute leukemia. *Blood* 1983 Aug;62(2):473-9.

[38]Bishop D, Tandy N, Anderson N, Bessos H, Seghatchian MJ. A clinical and laboratory study of platelet concentrates produced by pooled buffy coat and single donor apheresis technologies. *Transfus.Sci.* 1995 Jun;16(2):187-8.

[39]Kluter H, Dorges L, Maass E, Wagner T, Bartels H, Kirchner H. In-vivo evaluation of random donor platelet concentrates from pooled buffy coats. *Ann.Hematol.* 1996 Aug;73(2):85-9.

[40]Muylle L, Wouters E, Peetermans ME. Febrile reactions to platelet transfusion: the effect of increased interleukin 6 levels in concentrates prepared by the platelet-rich plasma method. *Transfusion* 1996 Oct;36(10):886-90.

[41]TRAP Study Group. Leukocyte reduction and ultraviolet B irradiation of platelets to prevent alloimmunization and refractoriness to platelet transfusions. The Trial to Reduce Alloimmunization to Platelets Study Group. *N.Engl.J.Med.* 1997 Dec 25;337(26):1861-9.

[42]Anderson NA, Gray S, Copplestone JA, Chan DC, Hamon M, Prentice AG, Johnson SA, Phillips M, van WG, Oakhill A, et al. A prospective randomized study of three types of platelet concentrates in patients with haematological malignancy: corrected platelet count increments and frequency of nonhaemolytic febrile transfusion reactions. *Transfus.Med.* 1997 Mar;7(1):33-9.

[43]Heddle NM, Blajchman MA, Meyer RM, Lipton JH, Walker IR, Sher GD, Constantini LA, Patterson B, Roberts RS, Thorpe KE, et al. A randomized controlled trial comparing the frequency of acute reactions to plasma-removed platelets and prestorage WBC-reduced platelets. *Transfusion* 2002 May;42(5):556-66.

[44]Enright H, Davis K, Gernsheimer T, McCullough JJ, Woodson R, Slichter SJ. Factors influencing moderate to severe reactions to PLT transfusions: experience of the TRAP multicenter clinical trial. *Transfusion* 2003 Nov;43(11):1545-52.

[45]Slichter SJ, Davis K, Enright H, Braine H, Gernsheimer T, Kao KJ, Kickler T, Lee E, McFarland J, McCullough J, et al. Factors affecting posttransfusion platelet increments, platelet refractoriness, and platelet transfusion intervals in thrombocytopenic patients. *Blood* 2005 May 15;105(10):4106-14.

[46]Heddle NM, Arnold DM, Boye D, Webert KE, Resz I, Dumont LJ. Comparing the efficacy and safety of apheresis and whole blood-derived platelet transfusions: a systematic review. *Transfusion* 2008 Jul;48(7):1447-58.

[47]Bishop JF, Matthews JP, Yuen K, McGrath K, Wolf MM, Szer J. The definition of refractoriness to platelet transfusions. *Transfus.Med.* 1992 Mar;2(1):35-41.

[48]Heddle NM, Klama L, Meyer R, Walker I, Boshkov L, Roberts R, Chambers S, Podlosky L, O'Hoski P, Levine M. A randomized controlled trial comparing plasma removal with white cell reduction to prevent reactions to platelets. *Transfusion* 1999 Mar;39(3):231-8.

[49]Arnold et al. A Randomized Crossover Trial to Compare *In Vivo* Recovery and Survival of Apheresis Platelets and Whole Blood Derived PLatelets in Health Volunteers. *Transfusion*. 2005. Ref Type: Abstract

[50]McFarland JG, Anderson AJ, Slichter SJ. Factors influencing the transfusion response to HLA-selected apheresis donor platelets in patients refractory to random platelet concentrates. *Br.J.Haematol.* 1989 Nov;73(3):380-6.

[51]Whitaker BI, Sullivan M. The 2005 Nationwide Blood Collection and Utilization: Survey Report. Rockville, MD: AABB, Bethesda MS and United States Department of Health and Human Services; 2005.

[52]America's blood centers: England bans FFP from female donors to prevent TRALI. ABC Newsl 2003:1-3.

In: Transfusion - Think About It
Editor: Trevor J. Cobain

ISBN 978-1-61668-969-8

Chapter 9

CLINICAL DECISION SUPPORT SYSTEMS: APPLICATIONS IN BLOOD TRANSFUSION

Leon L. Su
United Blood Services Arizona, Scottsdale, AZ, USA.

ABSTRACT

Computer based clinical decision support (CDS) systems are emerging as an important tool of modern health information systems. When thoroughly designed and tested, implementation of CDS systems can lead to reduced healthcare costs and improved outcomes in patient care. Today, the application of CDS to blood transfusion is in its infancy, and champions are needed to explore new opportunities. There are early reports of CDS applications in blood transfusion, many of which have primarily focused on the appropriate use of blood components. The ability of these systems to change transfusion practice is promising. As more hospitals begin to upgrade their health information infrastructure, CDS systems will become more available. This will lead to opportunities for transfusion medicine specialists to become involved in the development and implementation of CDS programs applied to blood transfusion. In time, CDS technology will likely play a significant role in the way medicine is practiced. With careful planning and evaluation, CDS has the potential to take transfusion practice to a safer and more effective level.

INTRODUCTION

There is no better time than the present for the transfusion medicine community to begin thinking of ways to bring clinical decision support (CDS) systems into the fold of transfusion practice. In recent years there has been intense interest from public and private sectors to apply computer based information systems, including tools such as CDS, the electronic medical record (EMR), and computerized physician order entry (CPOE), to healthcare. Collectively termed "information technology", the use of such technology is underutilized in healthcare as compared to other industries. The recognition that the healthcare industry is lagging in adopting new technology has spurred growing support for modernization of the healthcare industry with the intent of reducing healthcare costs and improving patient care.

Much of the interest to modernize healthcare stems from the medical errors that continue to impact patient safety and cost of care. In a 1999 report from the Institute of Medicine, it is estimated that up to a million injuries and 98,000 deaths occur each year as a direct result of medical errors [1]. Of equal concern is a report from the U.S. President's health information technology plan which states that as much as $300 billion is spent each year in the U.S. on treatments that are unnecessary, inappropriate or ineffective [2]. Problems such as poor coordination and communication, administrative inefficiencies and uncertain value of medical interventions all contribute to excess healthcare spending.

In an effort to change the landscape of healthcare in the U.S., the President of the United States signed an executive order back in April of 2004 announcing a commitment to develop a nationwide health information network. Within this order is a call for most Americans to have seamless and secure electronic health records within 10 years. To this end, a surge of federal initiatives have emerged to bring standardized health information systems to a national level. Over time, there is the expectation that this initiative and others similar to it in other parts of the world will begin to bridge the gap to a global health network and improve the way medicine is practiced. Until then, the immediate effect is that more healthcare organizations will begin to implement up-to-date health information systems, which in turn, will usher in CDS technology to more hospitals. It is at the early stages of implementation that many transfusion medicine experts can begin to explore and define a role for CDS in blood transfusion.

Overview of Clinical Decision Support Systems

CDS is defined as "providing clinicians or patients with clinical knowledge and patient-related information, intelligently filtered, or presented at appropriate times, to enhance patient care" [3]. Traditional forms of CDS, using means other than computers, have included paper-based order forms, manual auditing with feedback, and didactic education to providers. Modern CDS solutions greatly expand upon the capabilities of traditional CDS by relying on information technology to perform interventions. As a result, more sophisticated and functional CDS solutions have been developed using computer information systems.

It is expected that many of the gains seen with health care reform using information technology will come directly from the implementation of computer based CDS systems. Systematic reviews of studies to evaluate the effect of CDS systems on healthcare have shown promising benefits in the areas of drug dosing, practitioner performance, preventative care, disease management, regulatory compliance, and other aspects of medical care [4-8]. Reports of CPOE systems combined with CDS have been shown to reduce medication error rates anywhere from 55 to 83% [9,10] and improve overall outcomes such as survival, length of stay in hospitals, and cost of care [11-13]. Yet, not all CDS systems are created equal, and while some studies evaluating CDS implementation have shown benefit, other studies to date have failed to show clear benefits in overall patient outcomes. There are an impressive number of studies which show that adoption of CDS systems show no improvement in clinical practice [5]. While these studies may appear discouraging for CDS implementation, they serve a greater purpose in identifying which CDS components do and do not work in the clinical setting.

In a systematic review performed by Kawamoto and colleagues, a total of seventy studies investigating the ability of CDS to improve clinical practice were reviewed and decision support systems were seen to significantly improve clinical practice in 68% of the trials reviewed [14]. From these trials, several features of CDS systems were identified as independent predictors for improved clinical practice: systems that provide support automatically during workflow and at the time and place of decision making, systems that deliver support through computer technology, and systems that provide recommendations rather than assessments. These features, and other yet-to-be discovered CDS functions that demonstrate a positive impact on patient care, are the cornerstone for developing effective CDS solutions.

Computer-based CDS applications range from simple CDS with no inherent logic to more extensive solutions that provide decision support using multiple data sources and a complex logic system. The broad range of complexity and function seen in different CDS systems underscores the challenge in classifying CDS systems in the literature. The result is that there is currently no universally-accepted taxonomy to categorize CDS systems. In one report, CDS systems are categorized into 4 broad areas that can be supported by CDS; these include administrative tasks, managing clinical complexity and details, controlling costs, and decision support [15]. Alternatively, CDS systems can be organized by decision support function and examples include preventative care, event monitoring, ordering assistance, diagnosis support, and disease management. CDS applications can also be categorized by the type of intervention used. CDS interventions include reminders and alerts, specialized documentation forms, presentation of patient data and/or reference information at relevant times, custom order sets and choice lists, and intelligent systems to support drug dosing, diagnosis and disease management [3,4,14].

Overview of CDS design

The overall design of a CDS system may vary and change with new technology, but there are certain basic components that are common to most CDS interventions. At the heart of a CDS application is the inference engine (IE) which is responsible for processing the flow of data going in to and out of the CDS system. The IE executes logic which eventually results in an action leading to the CDS intervention; this can then be displayed to the user via a user interface. To perform its functions, the IE requires data, often in the form of knowledge bases and patient-related information. Patient-related information includes demographics, clinical data repositories, laboratory test results and other information linked to a specific patient [16,17]. Generally speaking, knowledge bases at its simplest form can consist of experienced-based knowledge from domain experts, textbook data, and evidence-based knowledge from clinical trials [17,18]. To create and maintain knowledge bases, knowledge engineers, who are experts in software development and CDS infrastructure, can work with domain experts (e.g. transfusion medicine specialist) to translate clinical knowledge into code that can be utilized by the IE. A unique type of knowledge base worth noting are medical logic modules (MLM) that are constructed with a programming language, standardized by Health Level Seven, known as Arden syntax [19]. These modules are designed to work independently from one another and contain sufficient knowledge and logic to perform a single medical decision. There are several advantages to using MLMs and Arden syntax in a CDS system. MLMs can be shared with other institutions reducing the need for each organization to recreate intervention algorithms that already exist. In addition, the target user for Arden syntax is the clinician or domain expert with little programming experience; hence it is more easily adopted by the experts who provide clinical knowledge. MLMs can be seamlessly imbedded into health information systems that are "Arden-compliant" and thus shared between institutions that have such systems. At the time this chapter was written, vendors with applications that are "Arden-compliant" included Eclipsys Corporation, McKesson Information Solutions, and Siemens Medical Solutions Health Services Corporation [20]. Institutions that currently have or plan to implement an information system from one of these companies can build their CDS solutions by either acquiring existing MLMs and modifying them for their institution or creating new MLMs using Arden Syntax. A dated set of MLMs already constructed can be found at a MLM library website through the Department of Medical Informatics at Columbia University [21]. In addition, vendors such as MICROMEDEX (Medical Logic Modules) have begun to offer commercial MLM packages that offer comprehensive CDS applications.

CDS in Blood Transfusion

CDS systems applied with extensive preparation and testing could have a great impact in improving outcomes of blood transfusion. Audits of blood transfusion products reported in the literature suggest that there is still misuse as well as over- and under-utilization of blood products in the hospital setting; thus resulting in added costs and a greater incidence of adverse effects and blood product wastage [22-26]. Contributing to the problem of blood product mismanagement is the observation that transfusion practices vary widely among clinicians, suggesting the need for additional clinical trials and improved utilization of evidence-based medicine to better define transfusion management strategies [18,27-29]. Innovative, computer-based CDS solutions aimed at the issues above have great potential in improving blood utilization and patient safety. Already proven to improve blood product utilization are behaviour interventions performed through manual audits, guidelines, education and specialized forms [30-35]. A systematic review of these behavioural interventions suggests that, as a whole, they are effective in modifying transfusion practices and optimizing blood utilization [36]. Delivery of behaviour interventions within a CDS system could likely further improve its effectiveness. In addition, CDS applications can improve outcomes in blood transfusion by improving compliance with regulatory guidelines. Similar to the external and internal quality measures which affect the operation of a hospital and drive CDS adoption, transfusion services are also subject to rigid, quality assurance guidelines that can benefit from CDS implementation.

Existing Applications of CDS to Support Blood Transfusion Practice

CDS systems applied to improving transfusion practice do exist in the literature, yet little is known about which systems work best in improving outcomes in blood transfusion. Of the systems reported, some solutions appear promising, while others fall short of making a significant impact in improving blood product utilization. Numerous studies have described the use of computer-based auditing to assess blood transfusion practices, and while these studies demonstrate how efficient prospective monitoring of blood transfusion can be using computer assistance, many of these systems only identify problem areas but fail to take any immediate action with audited information [37-40]. The majority of these systems have great potential in becoming more developed CDS applications in the form of event monitoring systems - a CDS function commonly utilized in health information systems. An event monitoring system would not only monitor blood transfusion practices as the systems above are capable of doing, but take it one step further and apply the audit information to knowledge bases to yield a conclusion. The conclusion could then be delivered to the clinician in the form of an alert, reminder, or specialized order list.

An excellent example of a CDS application that was designed to monitor blood transfusion orders and provide recommended feedback was a system developed by Rothschild and colleagues at the Brigham and Women's hospital [41]. In their design, evidence based guidelines were established beforehand and placed in knowledge databases. A CDS application was then designed and tied into the hospital's CPOE system. The system worked as follows: when ordering blood products, physicians would choose the blood component, dosage, and administration rate. Indications for the transfusion would then be selected from a predetermined list. If the order was determined urgent by the system, blood product orders would be processed immediately. In non-urgent situations, additional screens would request patient information and then CDS logic would compare the product order to the pre-established guidelines in the database. Deviations from guidelines would send recommendations immediately to the clinician, where a decision could then be made to accept or reject the CDS recommendations. A study of this CDS intervention was performed in 2003-2004 in a randomized controlled trial and showed a strikingly high percentage of inappropriate transfusion orders in 72% of house staff at baseline. Following CDS intervention, the percentage of inappropriate orders dropped to roughly 60%. Of the total CDS recommendations given, 14% of the recommended orders were accepted. In summary, the study demonstrated effectiveness of CDS in reducing inappropriate transfusions, but did not correlate this reduction with any improvement in transfusion outcomes.

Another example of a real world CDS application in blood transfusion is a system developed by Achour and colleagues that uses MLMs built with a specialized (Unified Medical Language System-based) knowledge acquisition tool [42]. In their report, multiple MLMs were created using rule sets that would help the clinician decide whether or not blood transfusion was needed and what blood products were appropriate to give. The CDS event could be triggered in one of two ways: either by data in the form of a new haemoglobin or platelet level which would then trigger an alert if the values were critical, or by the clinician seeking consultation at the time of blood product ordering. In the consultation mode, the physician enters data regarding the blood product order and other patient information, and the system then determines if blood transfusion is appropriate and makes recommendations on what blood products to give. The ordering physician then has the option to accept the recommendation or reject it and give a brief reason. Preliminary results from an evaluation of their system showed that the CDS system was highly reliable with regard to coherence and correctness of the intervention, but discrepancies were seen between the system and ordering physicians regarding the different types of specialized blood product to give [43].

Interestingly, modification of the MLMs did not resolve the discrepancy but when the orders were reviewed by a transfusion medicine expert, it was suggested that the discrepancy was not related to the CDS system, but rather, to ordering physicians that did not adhere to the same transfusion guidelines as the transfusion medicine specialists.

An interesting but not yet fully developed application of CDS in blood transfusion is a report of an artificial neural network medical decision support tool that accurately predicts the transfusion requirements of ER patients based on available data at presentation [44]. Evaluation of the system indicates that it can give a reliable prediction of transfusion needs and provide clinicians with helpful information to assist in patient management. However, like other reported applications of CDS in blood transfusion, further evaluation is needed to determine if such applications lead to improvements in transfusion outcomes and patient safety.

Identifying CDS Targets for Intervention

Reports of CDS systems in blood transfusion thus far have only begun to scratch the surface of what is possible. There are many potential areas that CDS can be used to improve outcomes in blood transfusion. Table 1 lists some widely-recognized problem areas in blood transfusion practice that may benefit from CDS.

Table 1. Problem areas in blood transfusion that may benefit from CDS

Inappropriate blood product ordering according to evidence-based medicine and/or local guidelines
▪ Over utilization/Misuse of a blood product in certain clinical situations ◦ pRBCs, Platelets, FFP, and/or Cryoprecipitate given in situations that do not meet predetermined criteria ◦ Ordering of specialized blood products (i.e. CMV-negative, irradiated, washed) without a proper indication ▪ Underutilization of a blood product in certain clinical situations ◦ Failure to order cryoprecipitate, fresh frozen plasma and platelets in a timely manner during massive transfusion ◦ Failure to order HLA-matched or cross-matched platelets in patients with immune-mediated platelet refractoriness ◦ Failure to order specialized blood products (i.e. CMV-negative, irradiated, washed) when indicated ▪ Correct blood product order for the given clinical situation but incorrect dosing
Non-compliance with regulatory guidelines
▪ Underreporting of post-transfusion adverse reactions

These problem areas make excellent targets for CDS for several reasons. First, as previously mentioned, the literature demonstrates that blood ordering and the reporting of post-transfusion adverse events are suboptimal, and there is a universal need to find and implement new solutions to improve these issues. Second, addressing these problems with CDS serves high-end institutional goals that drive CDS adoption, such as improving patient safety, providing more efficient patient care, and reducing costs. Lastly, these problems share in common the fact that they are all dependent on the provider's decision-making process, thus are theoretically correctable by CDS. While the list in table 1 provides a good starting point for developing CDS interventions aimed at improving outcomes in blood transfusion, there are many other possible goals and objectives that can be identified depending on the needs and local practice of the institution. The selection of additional goals and objectives requires a thorough understanding of how the end-users (clinicians and nurses) are involved with the process of blood transfusion (from ordering blood to post-transfusion follow-up). Any decision point along the continuum of blood product administration has the potential to be improved by CDS intervention.

Exploring CDS Solutions in Blood Transfusion

Once clinical targets have been selected for intervention, there are multiple CDS options that can be considered depending on an institution's information system infrastructure. In general, a CDS system can provide functional support in the form of preventative care, event monitoring, ordering assistance, diagnosis support, and disease management. Current commercial CDS programs applicable to blood transfusion practice mostly aim to improve blood product selection using a rules-based event monitoring system, an ordering assistance application, or a hybrid of the two. Again, these applications can monitor blood product orders, laboratory results, and/or other patient-related data, and then intervene when an inappropriate blood product order is identified.

Less explored solutions that have great potential in improving outcomes in blood transfusion may utilize other CDS functions such as preventative care, diagnosis support and disease management. In a preventative care system, CDS support can identify patients that need specialized blood products and recommend such products at the time of blood product ordering. Patients at greatest risk for complications of cytomegalovirus infection, graft versus host disease, severe allergic reactions, or alloimmunization to human leukocyte antigens can be identified by searching patient-related data prior to or at the time of blood product ordering. The intervention can then provide patient-specific order sets, or alternatively, display an alert or reference material to educate and guide the clinician into making the appropriate product choice.

CDS applications that provide diagnosis support can apply intelligent systems to areas such as dilutional coagulopathy in massive transfusion, immune-mediated platelet refractoriness, and post-transfusion adverse reactions. These intelligent systems can be more complex than an event monitoring system in that they analyze multiple patient data points over time and apply logic at each step in order to recognize the diagnosis. For instance, an information system with CDS support could identify massive transfusion situations from the frequency and timing of previous red blood cell orders and provide recommendations for frozen plasma and/or cryoprecipitate. The same system could also analyze blood counts and platelet transfusions and alert the clinician to a possible refractory patient with the recommendation for further tests and HLA- or cross-matched platelets.

Also worth noting is the potential for CDS systems to provide disease management support. Such solutions applicable to blood transfusion can utilize intelligent systems to predict transfusion requirements for different clinical situations. Algorithms predicting transfusion requirements for different clinical scenarios can be found in the literature and on the Internet [45-48]. An intelligent system that combines such algorithms and patient data could then provide real-time support to help manage different disease states requiring blood transfusion.

Role of the Transfusion Medicine Physician/Specialist in Blood Banking

CDS applications aimed at blood transfusion have the potential to conserve blood inventory, improve patient outcomes, reduce costs and enhance compliance with regulatory agencies. With the growing number of institutions beginning to introduce health information systems into their organization, CDS programs will become more prevalent over time. As a result, there are emerging opportunities for experts in transfusion medicine to be involved with the process of CDS implementation. The transfusion medicine physician and/or technical leader in the blood bank can play a vital role in CDS development and provide the necessary expertise to help select appropriate CDS interventions in blood transfusion. As a participant in CDS implementation, the expert in transfusion medicine should understand the overall structure of CDS applications and become familiar with all of the potential interventions available. In doing so, they are better able to advise whether or not CDS interventions aimed at improving outcomes in blood transfusion are feasible at his/her institution. Furthermore, they can help identify clinical goals to target, and in those goals, find relevance to the greater needs of the organization. An even greater role for the expert in transfusion medicine is to become a "champion" for their CDS program. As a "champion", they can serve as a bridge between CDS management, IT staff, and end-users. They essentially take on greater responsibility for the development of CDS interventions and work to address any issues pertaining to the design, testing, validation and implementation of CDS systems. A "champion" can help design rule-based logic with IT staff and create algorithms to predict and manage blood product usage. In addition, the expert in transfusion medicine has the unique perspective of both laboratory and clinical operations, and thus can provide guidance on how to best serve both areas with CDS tools. They can spend time with end-users to understand the impact of CDS interventions and they can also work with other participants or "champions" to create CDS solutions that affect multiple disciplines. Lastly, the expert in transfusion medicine can play a role in evaluating and validating CDS interventions related to blood transfusion. Once a CDS intervention goes live, the transfusion medicine specialist can participate in quality assurance by monitoring results and conducting user surveys. At the very minimum, most transfusion experts will be interested in measuring results since the issues pertinent to a hospital's transfusion committee will likely involve measuring outcomes from CDS interventions.

Barriers and Negative Outcomes to CDS Systems

Despite much of the success and potential of CDS systems to improve health care delivery, implementation of CDS and information technology in health care has been slow [49]. One significant barrier to date involves the cost of implementation. Adoption of an up-to-date health information system in general is associated with high costs since a transformation of the workplace is often required. This includes new equipment purchases, loss of productivity as a result of workflow disruption, and allocation of resources dedicated to all aspects of implementation [50]. Additionally, the return in investment often requires long periods to accrue and the majority of initial savings is first evident only to health care insurers or patients [51,52]. While pay-for-performance programs and other external funding sources are available to help subsidize the costs of implementing new technology, the costs of introducing a CDS system can be substantial and thus out of reach for some hospitals and physician offices.

Another barrier to CDS adoption is the difficulty of implementation. The diversity of information system applications on the market and the range of CDS options available make it challenging to identify the best strategic plan for CDS development. In addition, access and maintenance of knowledge bases remains a difficult issue to address and information is still limited on which clinical targets and interventions lead to positive, rather than negative, outcomes.

Also limiting is the reluctance of some providers to accept CDS technology, thereby blunting the effectiveness of this technology to improve transfusion practice. Issues often cited as reasons for provider resistance include trouble recognizing the value of a CDS system, the potential threat to professional autonomy, and the perception of increased liability if CDS advice is rejected [50,53]. Finally, consideration should be given to the possibility that CDS systems have the capacity to inadvertently cause harm if not properly designed and validated. Unintended medical errors associated with health technology are already reported in the literature [54,55], emphasizing the need for careful planning and evaluation.

CONCLUSION

As the healthcare industry continues to reach new milestones with implementation of health technology, the role of CDS systems will become clearer. Current evidence shows that many functions and attributes of CDS can lead to improved outcomes in patient safety and healthcare costs, while other features have proven to provide no benefit and even introduce new medical errors. Implementation of effective CDS is clearly a challenge and requires extensive planning and support from many key personnel including administrators and end-users. Some benefits from CDS may not outweigh the cost of implementation and adding some technologies may be excessive. Validation and continued monitoring is therefore essential to determine if CDS solutions are appropriate and accomplish the goals they were set out to achieve.

While CDS in blood transfusion practice has not been fully explored, there is great potential for CDS applications to improve outcomes in blood transfusion. Not only can CDS be used to improve blood utilization, but it can also be used to prevent complications associated with blood products, enhance diagnosis recognition related to blood transfusions, and help mange blood usage for different disease states. Upcoming CDS programs interested in improving outcomes in blood transfusion should consider expanding the current applications of CDS in blood transfusion to beyond blood utilization.

Reports of early CDS interventions applied to blood transfusion practice are promising, but further evaluation in the form of randomized control studies is needed. The next step in the process will be for more organizations to begin looking at how they can apply their information systems and CDS technology to improve transfusion practice. Continued growth and success in this area will require advocacy and involvement from the transfusion medicine community and the support of clinicians and hospital administrators.

REFERENCES

[1] Kohn LT, Corrigan JM, Donaldson MS. *To err is human: building a safer health system* [report]. Washington, DC: National Academy Press; 1999.

[2] Transforming Health Care: The President's Health Information Technology Plan. [document on the Internet]. The White House; 2004 [cited 2008 August 26]. Available from: http://www.whitehouse.gov/infocus/technology/economic_policy200404/chap3.html

[3] Osheroff JA, Pifer EA, Teich JM, Sittig DF, Jenders RA. *Improving outcomes with clinical decision support: An Implementer's Guide*. Chicago (IL): HIMSS; 2005

[4] Garg AX, Adhikari NK, McDonald H, Rosas-Arellano MP, Devereaux PJ, Beyene J, Sam J, Haynes RB. Effects of Computerized Clinical Decision Support Systems on Practitioner Performance and Patient Outcomes: A Systematic Review. *JAMA*. 2005;293:1223-38.

[5] Hunt DL, Haynes RB, Hanna SE, Smith K. Effects of Computer-Based Clinical Decision Support Systems on Physician Performance and Patient Outcomes: A Systematic Review. *JAMA*. 1998;280(15):1339-46.

[6] Shea S, DuMouchel W, Bahamonde L. A meta-analysis of 16 randomized controlled trials to evaluate computer-based clinical reminder systems for preventative care in the ambulatory setting. *J Am Med Inform Assoc*. 1996;3:399-409.

[7] Kaushal R, Shojania KG, Bates DW. Effects of Computerized Physician Order Entry and Clinical Decision Support Systems on Medication Safety: A Systematic Review. *Arch Intern Med*. 2003;163:1409-16.

[8] Balas EA, Austin SM, Mitchell JA. The clinical value of computerized information services: a review of 98 randomized clinical trials. *Arch Fam Med*. 1996;5:271-8.

[9] Bates DW, Leape LL, Cullen DJ, Laird N, Petersen LA, Teich JM, Burdick E, Hickey M, Kleefield S, Shea B, Vander Vliet M, Seger DL. Effect of computerized physician order entry and a team intervention on prevention of serious medication errors. *JAMA*. 1998;280(15):1311-6.

[10] Bates DW, Miller EB, Cullen DJ, Burdick L, Williams L, Laird N, Petersen LA, Small SD, Sweitzer BJ, Vander Vliet M, Leape LL. Patient risk factors for adverse drug events in hospitalized patients. *Arch Intern Med*. 1999;159:2553-660.

[11] Evans RS, Pestotnik SL, Classen DC, Clemmer TP, Weaver LK, Orme JF Jr, Lloyd JF, Burke JP. A computer-assisted management program for antibiotics and other anti-infective agents. *N Engl J Med*. 1998;338:232-8.

[12] Rind D, Safran C, Phillips RS, Wang Q, Calkins DR, Delbanco TL, Bleich HL, Slack WV. Effect of computer-based alerts on the treatment and outcomes of hospitalized patients. *Arch Intern Med*. 1994;154:1511-7.

[13] Bates DW, Cohen M, Leape LL, Overhage JM, Shabot MM, Sheridan T. Reducing the frequency of errors in medicine using information technology. *J Am Med Inform Assoc*. 2001;8:299-308.

[14]Kawamoto K, Houlihan CA, Balas EA, Lobach DF. Improving clinical practice using clinical decision support systems: a systematic review of trials to identify features critical to success. *BMJ.* 2005;330:765-72.

[15]Perreault L, Metzger J. A pragmatic framework for understanding clinical decision support. *J Healthcare Info Management.* 1999.

[16]Sittig, DF. Prerequisites for a real-time clinical decision support system. The Informatics Review [serial online]. 1999 [cited 2008 August 26]. Available from: http://www.informatics-review.com/thoughts/prereqs.html.

[17]Mendonça EA, Jenders R, Lussier YA. Clinical decision support systems. In: Beaver K, editor. *Healthcare Information Systems. second edition.* Boca Raton (FL): CRC Press; 2003. p. 221-35.

[18]Sim I, Gorman P, Greenes RA, Haynes RB, Kaplan B, Lehmann H, Tang PC. Clinical decision support systems for the practice of evidence-based medicine. *J Am Med Inform Assoc.* 2001;8:527-34.

[19]Hripcsak G, Ludemann P, Pryor TA, Wigertz OB, Clayton PD. Rationale for the Arden syntax. *Comput Biomed Res.* 1994;27(4):291-324.

[20]Jenders RA. The Arden syntax for medical logic systems [document on the Internet]. Health Level Seven, Inc; [updated 2006 July 21; cited 2008 August 26]. Available from: http://cslxinfmtcs.csmc.edu/hl7/arden/.

[21]CPMC Medical Logic Module Library [document on the Internet]. Columbia University; [updated 1997 March; cited 2008 August 26]. Available from: http://www.dmi.columbia.edu/resources/arden/mlm/cpmc-mlm-index.html.

[22]Goodnough LT, Soegiarso RW, Birkmeyer JD, Welch HG. Economic impact of inappropriate blood transfusions in coronary artery graft surgery. *Am J Med.* 1993;94:509-14.

[23]Khanna MP, Hébert PC, Fergusson DA. Review of the clinical practice literature on patient characteristics associated with perioperative allogeneic red blood cell transfusion. *Transfus Med Rev.* 2003;17(2):110-9.

[24]Schofield WN, Rubin GL, Dean MG. Appropriateness of platelet, fresh frozen plasma and cryoprecipitate transfusion in New South Wales public hospitals. *Med J Aust.* 2003;178(3):117-21.

[25]Chang H, Hawes H, Hall GA, Fuller K, Francombe WH, Zuber E, Sher GD. Prospective audit of cytomegalovirus-negative blood product utilization in haematology/oncology patients. *Transfus Med.* 1999;9(3):195-8.

[26]Pantanowitz L, Kruskall M, Uhl L. Cryoprecipitate Patterns of Use. *Am J Clin Pathol.* 2003;119:874-81.

[27]Stover EP, Siegal LC, Parks R, Levin J, Body SC, Maddi R, D'Ambra MN, Mangano DT, Spiess BD. Variability in transfusion practice for coronary artery disease persists despite national consensus guidelines: a 24 institution study. *Anesthesiology.* 1998;88:327-33.

[28]Wong EC, Perez-Albuerne E, Moscow JA, Luban NL. Transfusion management strategies: A survey of practicing pediatric hematology/oncology specialists. *Pediatr Blood Cancer.* 2005;44:119-27.

[29]Goodnough LT, Johnston MF, Toy PT. The variability in transfusion practice in coronary artery bypass surgery. *JAMA* .1991;265:86-90.

[30]Tuckfield A, Haeusler MN, Grigg AP, Metz J. Reduction of inappropriate use of blood products by prospective monitoring of transfusion request forms. *MJA.* 1997;167:473-6.

[31]Toy PT. The transfusion audit as an educational tool. *Transfu Sci.* 1998;19(1):91-6.
[32]Toy PT. Audit and education in transfusion medicine. *Vox Sang.* 1996;70(1):1-5.
[33]Mallett SV, Peachey TD, Sanehi O, Hazlehurst G, Mehta A. Reducing red blood cell transfusion in elective surgical patients: the role of audit and practice guidelines. *Anaesthesia.* 2000;55(10):1013-9.
[34]Toy PT. Guiding the decision to transfuse. *Arch Pathol Lab Med.* 1999;123:592-4.
[35]Hui CH, Williams I, Davis K. Clinical audit of the use of fresh-frozen plasma and platelets in a tertiary teaching hospital and the impact of a new transfusion request form. *Internal Medicine Journal.* 2005;35:283-8.
[36]Tinmouth A, MacDougall L, Fergusson D, Amin M, Graham ID, Hebert PC, Wilson K. Reducing the amount of blood transfused: A systematic review of behavioral interventions to change physicians' transfusion practices. *Arch Intern Med.* 2005;165:845-52.
[37]Hoeltge GA, Brown JC, Herzig RH, Johannisson MR, Millward BL, O'Hara PJ, Orlowski JP, Sharp DE, Zurick AM. Computer-assisted audits of blood component transfusion. *Cleve Clin J Med.* 1989;56(3):267-72.
[38]Kern DA, Bennett ST. Informatics applications in blood banking. *Clin Lab Med.* 1996;16(4):947-60.
[39]Petaja J, Anderson S, Syrjala M. A simple automatized audit system for following and managing practices of platelet and plasma transfusions in a neonatal intensive care unit. *Transfus Med.* 2004;14(4):281-8.
[40]Grey DE, Smith V, Villanueva G, Richards B, Augustson B, Erber WN. The utility of an automated electronic system to monitor and audit transfusion practice. *Vox Sang.* 2006;90(4):316-24.
[41]Rothschild JM, McGurk S, Honour M, Lu L, McClendon AA, Srivastava P, Churchill WH, Kaufman RM, Avorn J, Cook EF, Bates DW. Assessment of education and computerized decision support interventions for improving transfusion practice. *Transfusion.* 2007;47:228-39.
[42]Achour SL, Dojat M, Rieux C, Bierling P, Lepage E. Knowledge acquisition environment for the design of a decision support system: application in blood transfusion. *Proc AMIA Symp.* 1999:187-91.
[43]Achour SL, Dojat M, Rieux C, Bierling P, Lepage E. A UMLS-based Knowledge Acquisition Tool for Rule-based Clinical Decision Support System Development. *J AM Med Inform Assoc.* 2001;8:351-60.
[44]Walczak S. Artificial neural network medical decision support tool: predicting transfusion requirements of ER patients. *IEEE Trans Inf Technol Biomed.* 2005;9(3):468-74.
[45]The Medical Algorithms Project, Transfusion Medicine Chapter 5 [document on the Internet]. Institute for Algorithmic Medicine; 2007 January [cited 2008 August 26]. Available from: http://www.medal.org/visitor/www/active/ch5/ch5.aspx.
[46]Weber RS. A model for predicting transfusion requirements in head and neck surgery. *Laryngoscope.* 1995;105(73):1-17.
[47]Lacocque BJ, Gilbert K, Brien WF. Prospective validation of a point score system for predicting blood transfusion following hip or knee replacement. *Transfusion.* 1998;38:932-7.

[48]Wells PS. Safety and efficacy of methods for reducing perioperative allogeneic transfusions: a critical review of the literature. *Am J Ther*. 2002;9:377-88.
[49]Ash JS, Gorman PS, Seshadri V, Hersh WR. Computerized physician order entry in U.S. hospitals: results of a 2002 survey. *J Am Med Inform Assoc*. 2004;11(2):95-9.
[50]Ford EW, Menachemi N, Phillips MT. Predicting the adoption of electronic health records by physicians: when will health care be paperless? *J Am Med Inform Assoc*. 2006;13:106-12.
[51]Bolster C. National health IT initiative moves into action: an interview with David Brailer. *Healthcare Finan Manag*. 2005;59:92-3.
[52]Leatherman S, Berwick D, Iles D, Lewin LS, Davidoff F, Nolan T, Bisognano M. The business case for quality: case studies and an analysis. *Health Affairs*. 2003;22:17-30.
[53]Teich JM, Osheroff JA, Pifer EA, Sittig DF, Jenders RA. Clinical decision support in electronic prescribing: recommendations and an action plan [policy paper on the internet]. AMIA; 2005 March [cited 2008 August 26]. Available from: http://www.amia .org/mbrcenter/pubs/docs/cdswhitepaperforhhs-final2005-03-08.pdf.
[54]Koppel R, Metlay JP, Cohen A, Abaluck B, Localio AR, Kimmel SE, Strom BL. Role of computerized physician order entry systems in facilitating medication errors. *JAMA*. 2005;293(10):1197-203.
[55]Nebeker JR, Hoffman JM, Weir CR, Bennett CL, Hurdle JF. High rates of adverse drug events in a highly computerized hospital. *Arch Intern Med*. 2005;165(10):1111-6.

In: Transfusion - Think About It
Editor: Trevor J. Cobain
ISBN 978-1-61668-969-8

Chapter 10

THE VALUE OF RISK MODELLING TO SUPPORT BLOOD SAFETY POLICY DECISIONS

Clive R. Seed
Australian Red Cross Blood Service, Perth, Australia;
School of Surgery, University of Western Australia, Nedlands, Australia.

ABSTRACT

The contamination of blood supplies in France and Canada by HIV in the 1980's resulted in a severe loss of public confidence in blood transfusion worldwide. The ensuing focus by Governments on establishing 'Zero' risk blood supplies has lead to the incremental implementation of donor screening strategies in the form of new tests and donor deferrals. Each additional measure leads to a shrinking pool of eligible donors and places increasing pressure on the sufficient supply of blood and blood products.

Balancing the risk of safety and sufficiency is complex. One useful risk assessment tool is mathematical modelling increasingly used within the blood sector to estimate the risk associated with specific interventions. In this chapter two 'case studies' are used to illustrate the value of robust risk modelling to inform blood safety decision making.

The first considers the threat posed to the Australian blood supply from variant Creutzfeldt-Jakob (vCJD) disease. A mathematical model was developed to quantitate the then theoretical risk of vCJD transmission from a blood donor and compare it with the predicted increase in incidence of known pathogens resulting from the need to recruit an additional 50,000 first time donors, who are known to have higher viral incidence rates. The latter risk was associated with a proposed new donor deferral strategy which would indefinitely defer donors who had resided in the UK for a cumulative period of 6 months or more within the risk period. The model output indicated that the risk of vCJD transmission by blood was greater than that from the additional recruitment of first time donors and this data informed the eventual Australian policy decision to implement a vCJD deferral for residence in the UK.

The second case considers the strategy of testing donors at risk of malaria exposure and re-instating them for cellular component production earlier than the original deferral period. This strategy delivers a significant efficiency gain in terms of cellular blood components but potentially increases the risk of transfusion transmitted malaria. A mathematical model was developed to quantitate the risk differential between the existing deferral for 1-3 years versus deferral for a minimum period of 4 months with subsequent malaria antibody screening. The model predicted a negligible risk increase of 1 in 6 million for a transmission involving *P. falciparum*, the most important species in terms of recipient mortality. This novel risk modelling provided important evidence supporting the eventual implementation of a malaria antibody testing strategy in Australia.

INTRODUCTION

Invariably protecting the blood supply from both proven and potentially transfusion transmitted pathogens is a complex process which must balance the community's expectation of 'zero risk' against finite and competing financial resources with a receding number of eligible donors. Because one of the primary interventions generally applied against novel pathogens in advance of an appropriate test is exclusion of donors from identified risk groups (e.g. the widely applied vCJD donor deferral for residence in the UK) this balance can perhaps be likened to a pendulum which oscillates between 'sufficiency' and 'safety' of the blood supply.

Prior to the discovery of transmission of HIV and HCV by contaminated blood products in the early 1990's, this pendulum arguably favoured sufficiency. However the public's confidence in the safety of the blood supply was severely shaken in the wake of the HIV contamination scandals in France and Canada resulting in a paradigm shift toward safety [1,2]. Government policy makers and their regulatory authorities subsequently favoured decisions based on the 'precautionary principle' founded on the concept that '....for situations of scientific uncertainty, the possibility of risk should be taken into account in the absence of proof to the contrary' [3]. The precautionary principle evolved as a policy standard of the European Environment Agency who, in 1992 published the following descriptive statement [4];

'In order to protect the environment, a precautionary approach should be widely applied, meaning that where there are threats of serious irreversible damage to the environment, lack of full scientific certainty should not be used as a reason for postponing cost-effective measures to prevent environmental degradation'.......

'The precautionary principle permits a lower level of proof of harm to be used in policy-making whenever the consequences of waiting for a higher level of proof may be *very costly and/or irreversible* (emphasis added).

Moreno [5] points out the significance of the genesis of the precautionary principle stating that '....the original context was environmentalism, where ecologic complexities and uncertainties present risks that, for all intents and purposes, may truly be inestimable and irreversible. Those conditions may not apply in other policy contexts.' He further argues that '...the misinterpretation has been to suppose that precautionism requires that only zero risk is acceptable, or at least something quite close to zero risk. Even advocates of the principle would recognise these subtle shifts in thinking as errors. In particular, it is clear that any decision has opportunity costs. The opportunity costs in the blood industry are, among others, the loss of many usable units of blood and the alienation of potential donors'......

Irrespective of the applicability of the precautionary principle to blood policy making, it has become the default standard for Governments in developed countries at least. This has invariably led to extreme pressure on blood services to maintain a sufficient donor base as each successive safety intervention reduces the number of eligible blood donors. Paradoxically, the resulting potential inability to meet demand for blood products must itself be considered a risk, should the shortage become severe enough. This highlights the need to underpin blood policy decisions with 'evidence based' risk assessments utilising the best available data and expertise. Doing so provides the opportunity to properly assess the impact of competing risks, including the risk to sufficiency.

One useful risk assessment tool is mathematical modelling increasingly used within the blood sector to estimate the risk associated with specific interventions. In this chapter two 'case studies' are used to illustrate the value of robust risk modelling both in a predictive manner to inform blood safety policy decisions, and retrospectively to validate decisions or derive residual risk estimates for viral pathogens.

Case Study 1 - Validating the Australian Donor Deferral Policy for Variant Creutzfeldt-Jakob (vCJD) Disease

The finding in the mid 1990's that a significant number of plasma pools used to manufacture therapeutic protein derivatives contained donations from individuals who had subsequently died from classical Creutzfeldt-Jakob (CJD) disease resulted in concern over potential transmission of the infectious agent by these products. The laboratory experimental evidence at the time indicated that at least in rodent models low levels of infectivity were present in blood during the incubation and clinical phases of disease although this has never been confirmed [6]. Regulators variously responded by issuing guidance on whether to quarantine/recall affected lots. For example, in 1995 the US FDA introduced product recall measures when a donor included in a plasma pool was discovered to be at risk of classical CJD. Plasma product recalls continued in both Europe and the US until 1998 when the FDA withdrew its recall policy in consideration of widespread epidemiological evidence of the lack of classical CJD cases in long term blood product recipients and experimental demonstration of the removal of prions by the plasma fractionation process [7].

The 1996 discovery in the UK of a new 'variant' form of CJD (vCJD) associated with the ingestion of foodstuffs contaminated with the putative agent causing bovine spongiform encephalopathy (BSE) lead to similar concerns about the potential for transmission from blood and blood products. Despite the lack of transfusion associated case of vCJD at the time evidence from sheep infection studies demonstrated the potential for transmission of vCJD from blood [8]. In response the UK Department of Health commissioned a risk assessment of the theoretical risk of transfusion transmission of vCJD by blood which recommended certain steps designed to minimise this risk [9]. These steps included; the replacement from overseas of all UK-derived plasma for fractionation and the implementation of universal leukodepletion for donated blood. Both of these recommendations were implemented in 1999 by the UK National Blood Service [10].

In the absence of a suitable test and based on the initial observation that cases of vCJD were largely confined to UK residents, blood services worldwide began considering deferral of donors resident in the UK. The exact form of the deferral varied but generally it required that donors be indefinitely deferred if they had spent a cumulative period of 3 to 6 months or more in the UK between 1980 and 1996, the period considered to constitute the risk of acquiring vCJD.

Development of an Australian Deferral Policy

Considering the merits of instituting a deferral to minimise the then 'theoretical' risk that vCJD might be transmitted by blood transfusion was both complex and challenging. It constitutes an excellent case study in balancing several safety risks with the ultimate aim of minimising the overall risk exposure to blood recipients. These risks include;

1. The risk to sufficiency associated with the loss of donors/donations
2. The risk of transfusion transmitted vCJD associated with collecting blood from an asymptomatic donor incubating vCJD
3. The risk of an increased incidence of known infectious pathogens (HIV, HCV and HBV) resulting from the requirement to recruit an increased proportion of 'first' time donors (proven to have a higher incidence of 'recent' infection) to replace deferred repeat donors.

Although there was insufficient time to complete a formal risk assessment prior to government action, the completed risk assessment was coordinated by the ARCBS and subsequently published [11]. In mid-2000 a government decision was taken to implement a new donor deferral for cumulative time spent in the UK which was subsequently implemented in December. Nonetheless, components of the risk assessment were available at the time of the decision and therefore informed the eventual policy. It is informative to consider the individual risks and in particular the data and analysis undertaken to compare estimates of risks associated with proven versus theoretical transfusion transmitted pathogens.

Risk 1- Estimated Loss of Donors/Donations

Method

In order to estimate the donor loss ARCBS conducted a survey of the travel histories of its 1998 donor base (table 1).

Results

The 1998 ARCBS travel survey found that 20.7% of blood donations were made by donors who had visited the UK for less than 3 months between 1980 and 1996, and 8.3% of donations from donors who had visited for more than 3 months. Of these, 5.3% of donations were from donors who had visited for more than six months, and 3.6% of donations were from donors who had stayed for more than 12 months. In 1998 a total of 946,000 blood donations were made in Australia. Excluding donations from donors who had lived in the UK for six months or more (the eventual policy) would represent a loss of 50,100 donations from the blood supply in 1998 [11].

Table 1. Duration of residence in UK of Australian blood donors based on 1998 ARCBS survey

Duration residence in UK (months)	Assumed average duration of residence within strata (months)	Percentage of donations
0-1	0.5	12.9%
1-2	1.5	5.5%
2-3	2.5	2.3%
3-4	3.5	1.6%
4-5	4.5	1.1%
5-6	5.5	0.7%
6-12	9	1.7%
12+	36	3.6%

Reproduced with permission from reference 11.

Risk 2- Estimates of the Annual Number of Donations in Australia from Asymptomatic vCJD Infected Blood Donors

Method

In order to estimate the potential for asymptomatic carriage of vCJD in Australia, data from the epidemic in the UK were extrapolated to the Australian donor population based on the 1998 travel data as described by Correll et al [11].

1. Reported diagnoses and estimated total numbers of vCJD cases in UK

The UK National CJD Surveillance Unit reported in January 2001 that there had been 32 confirmed or probable vCJD cases in the UK in 2000, compared with 15 for the whole of 1999 [12]. Ghani et al [12] modelled estimates of the total number of people infected with and likely to develop vCJD in the future in the UK using vCJD mortality rates. The total number of vCJD-infected people in the UK was estimated to be between 63 and 136,000 cases. These estimates were dependent on the incubation period of vCJD and the pattern of future vCJD-diagnoses in the UK.

2. Estimates of the annual number of donations in Australia from asymptomatic vCJD infected blood donors

Estimates of the number of blood donations from asymptomatic donors infected with vCJD were made in following way. First, the prevalence of asymptomatic vCJD infection in UK residents, including lower and upper limits, was obtained from the modelled estimates of total numbers of people with vCJD [12]. Duration of exposure of UK residents to vCJD was taken to be 10 years between 1980 and 1996, reflecting the protective measures taken in the late 1980s and early 1990s. Second, vCJD prevalence among blood donors in Australia was assumed to be the same as that in the UK, but was assumed to be proportional to the duration of time spent in the UK. Details of the duration lived in the UK used in these analyses, and the assumed average durations lived in the UK within each strata, are given in Table 1. For example, prevalence of vCJD in blood donors who had lived in the UK for between 6 and 12 months between 1980 and 1996 was taken to be 7.5% (9/120 months) of the estimated prevalence of vCJD in UK residents. Upper and lower limits on these estimates were obtained based on the upper and lower limits of total vCJD prevalence in UK residents.

Results

1. Reported diagnoses and estimated total numbers of vCJD cases in UK

Given that there were 32 cases in 2000, reported to 3 January 2001, the estimates used in the Australian analysis were based on there being an average incidence of vCJD diagnoses in the UK of more than 15 cases per year in 2000-2002. Assuming at least 15 vCJD diagnoses annually in the UK between 2000-2002, the total number of vCJD infected people was estimated by Ghani et al [12] to be in the range 105 to 136,000 cases. In the Australian analyses, the number of vCJD infected people in the UK resident population was taken to be in the range 100 to 136,000, with a best estimate of 5,000 taken arbitrarily as the rough mid-point of this range (on a logarithm base 10 scale). This range of estimates was consistent with estimates of vCJD prevalence based on results of testing stored tonsil and appendix biopsies in the UK [12,13]. Based on the 1997 UK resident population of 58,726,000 people, these estimates correspond to a prevalence of vCJD-infection in the UK of 85 per million (range 2 to 2,300 per million).

2. Estimates of the annual number of donations in Australia from asymptomatic vCJD infected blood donors

Australia wide, it was estimated that in 1998 the annual total number of blood donations made by donors infected with vCJD was 1.15 (with a range, based on the uncertainty in the UK prevalence estimate, of 0.02 to 31.1). It was estimated that excluding donors who had spent more than six months in the UK would have resulted in the removal in 1998 of 0.92 donations per year that came from donors with vCJD (limits: 0.04 to 25.05 donations per year). The number of donations from vCJD infected donors was estimated to be slightly lower if donors who had spent more than a year in the UK were excluded (0.85, range 0.03-23.08), and slightly higher if donors who had spent 3 months or more were excluded (1.01, range 0.04 to 27.49).

Risk 3 - Increased risks of HIV, HCV and HBV infected donations donated during the window period

Method

To estimate the additional risk incurred by increasing the proportion of first time donors in the donor base as a result of deferring repeat donors, a separate risk estimate for each donor status was required. Since published models at the time of the risk assessment, including the most widely applied Incidence/Window period [14] model did not allow for this, their application was problematic. In light of this a novel model was developed to separately estimate the risk of a donation being infected with HIV, HCV or HBV, and being donated during the corresponding window period for both first time and repeat donors [11].

These risks were calculated from estimates of:

- the window periods for nucleic acid testing (NAT) for HIV and HCV [15] introduced to screen donated blood in Australia in June 2000
- the serological window period for HBsAg testing [16]

- the median interval between donations for repeat donors who seroconverted in 1998
- the average duration of infection for a person infected with each virus
- estimates of prevalence of each virus in first time and repeat donors in Australia

For first time donors, the risk of a donation from an infected donor being donated within the window period was calculated as the window period duration divided by the average lifetime duration of infection. For repeat donors, the risk of a donation from an infected donor being donated within the window period was calculated as the window period duration divided by the average time between repeat donations, which assumes that the negative test result for the previous blood donation was truly negative. For both first time and repeat donors, these probabilities were then multiplied by the probability of a single donation being from an infected donor (i.e. prevalence of infection in first time and repeat donors) to give the overall risk per donation. To allow for uncertainties in the median interval between donations for repeat donors who seroconverted in 1998, and the average duration of infection for a person infected with each virus, upper and lower limits were specified for each of these parameters. These specified limits were used to calculate upper and lower plausible limits on the risk of a donation being from an infected donor and donated within a window period for both first time and repeat donors. These plausible ranges should not be interpreted as confidence intervals, but rather as sensitivity analyses aimed at giving a notion of the uncertainties in final estimates associated with the assumptions made regarding these parameters.

Model Definitions

First Time Donor (FTD).

A first time donor is a donor who has not previously attended to donate.

Repeat Donor (RD)

A repeat donor is a donor who has a previously recorded attendance as a donor.

Window Period (WP)

The time between infection and first detection of the viral marker (unique to each test).

Seroconverter

A donor considered to have 'seroconverted' for an agent if prior to their seropositive donation they had made a previous 'negative' donation using a test of comparable. sensitivity

Prevalence of first-time donations (p(FTD))

The rate of confirmed seropositive donations per million first-time donations.

Prevalence of repeat donations (p(RD))

The rate of confirmed seropositive donations per million repeat donations.

Median Pre-seroconversion interval (I)

Median interval in days between the seropositive and seronegative donations for all seroconverters.

Average Life Time Risk (LTR)

The average lifetime infection duration in days. Based on the viral epidemiology and primary modes of transmission in Australia LTR's were assigned as HCV 9125 days (25 years), HBV 3,650 days (10 years) and HIV 3650 days (10 years).

Repeat Donor Risk calculation

$$P\ (RD) = WP/I \times p(RD)$$

First Time Donor Risk calculation

$$P\ (FTD) = WP/LTR \times p(FTD)$$

Total donor population risk

$$P\ (\text{total donor population}) = \text{FTD proportion} \times P(FTD) + \text{RD proportion} \times P(RD)$$

The model was initially used to provide background estimates of the risk of HIV, HCV or HBV infected donations being made during the relevant window periods. Estimates of the risks of infected donations being made during the window period were then made for each virus under three scenarios: first a best estimate scenario in which 33% of replacement donations were from first time donors and 67% from repeat donations; second a more conservative scenario in which 50% of replacement donations were from first time donors and 50% from repeat donations; and third a most conservative scenario in which all replacement donations were obtained from first time donors. Estimates of the increased risk of infected window period donations due to increased donor deferral were then made for each scenario by subtracting the current estimated background risk. Again, upper and lower plausible limits were calculated based on the ranges calculated for the risks of infected donations from first time and repeat donors described above.

Results

In 1998, first-time donors made up 12.1% of the donor population in Australia. However, in 1998 first-time donors contributed 5 of the 6 (83%) blood donations found to be infected with HIV, 209 of the 228 (92%) donations infected with HCV, and 133 of the 143 (93%) donations infected with HBV, which were detected through screening blood donations. The risks of a single blood donation being made by a donor infected with HIV, HCV or HBV, and donated during the relevant window period for HIV, HBV and HCV, with upper and lower plausible ranges, are summarised in Table 2. For HIV, the estimated risks of a blood donation being infected and donated during the window period were 1 in 7.6 million for first time donors and 1 in 32.9 million for repeat donors. For HCV the risks were 1 in 220,000 and 1 in 400,000 for first time and repeat donors respectively, and for HBV, 1 in 53,000 and 1 in 760,000 for new and repeat donors respectively.

If donors who had spent more than six months in the UK were deferred, the number of replacement HIV-infected donations being donated during the window period for HIV was estimated to increase by 0.0010 (plausible range 0.0007 to 0.0014) per year if 33% of donations were replaced with first time donors, by 0.0019 (0.0012 to 0.0026) per year if 50% of donations were replaced with first time donors, and 0.0044 (0.0028 to 0.0059) per year if all donations were replaced with first time donors. For HCV the number of infected donations made during a window period was estimated to increase by 0.021 (0.003 to 0.97), 0.038 (0.006 to 0.068) and 0.089 (0.014 to 0.157) donations per year for 33%, 50% and 100% replacement of donations by first time donors respectively, and for HBV, the increase was

0.18 (0.08 to 0.38), 0.33 (0.15 to 0.68) and 0.76 (0.33 to 1.57) donations per year respectively.

Table 2. Calculating the risk of infected donations during the window period[a]

	HIV	HCV	HBV
Window period for nucleic acid testing (NAT) - antigen testing for HBV (days)	11	23	59
Median interval between donations among 1998 repeat donors who had seroconverted (days)	436 *(500, 300)*	208 *(250, 150)*	539 *(600, 400)*
Estimated duration of infection (years)	10 *(12, 8)*	25 *(30, 20)*	10 *(20, 5)*
Risk of new donors being infected but missed by screening	1 in 7,600,000 *(1 in 6,100,000, 1 in 9,100,000)*	1 in 220,000 *(1 in 170,000, 1 in 260,000)*	1 in 53,000 *(1 in 28,000, 1 in 107,000)*
Risk of repeat donors being infected but missed by screening	1 in 32,900,000 *(1 in 22,700,000, 1 in 37,800,000)*	1 in 400,000 *(1 in 290,000 1 in 480,000),*	1 in 760,000 *(1 in 560,000, 1 in 840,000)*

a. Figures given in parentheses are lower and upper plausible limits
Reproduced with permission from reference 11.

Evaluating the Relative Risks

The potential loss of more than 50,000 donations per annum representing more than 5% of collections was undeniably a serious sufficiency risk. However, contingency measures including increased recruitment were available to mitigate the risk and based on previous experience in Australia had a high likelihood of success.

Given this, the outcome of the Australian risk assessment primarily depended on the relative magnitude of the risk to the blood supply posed directly from donors incubating vCJD versus the indirect risk of increasing the likelihood of collecting blood from a donor in the window period for HIV, HCV or HBV infection. The modelling indicated that excluding donors based on six months cumulative time spent in the UK between 1980 and 1996 would result in the exclusion of approximately one blood donation per year from an asymptomatic donor potentially infected with vCJD, though the upper limit on this estimate was as high as 25 donations per year from vCJD infected donors. In comparison, if donations from donors who had lived in the UK for more than six months between 1980 and 1996 were excluded, and if as predicted 33% of excluded donations were replaced by donations from first time donors, then the increase in window period donations per annum was estimated to be approximately 0.001 (1 donation every one thousand years) for HIV, 0.021 (1 donation every 50 years) for HCV, and 0.183 (1 donation every 5 years) for HBV. The overall risk increase therefore (summing the individual risks) was 0.2041 HIV, HCV or HBV WP donations per annum, less than the comparative figure of 0.92 potentially infectious vCJD donations.

Modelling by definition requires certain assumptions leading to caveats on these estimates. Importantly, at the time the transmissibility of vCJD through blood transfusion in humans was not established, even though it had been shown that it was possible for transmission to occur by this route in sheep [8]. The risk of transmitting vCJD through blood donations from donors with vCJD was therefore a theoretical rather than an actual risk. There was also substantial uncertainty in the overall prevalence of vCJD in UK residents, which lead to large uncertainties as to the likely prevalence of asymptomatic vCJD infection in blood donors in Australia who have lived in the UK. Estimates of the likely vCJD prevalence in UK residents adopted at the time of the analyses were based on modelled projections of vCJD mortality in UK residents who have a susceptible genotype. It was conceivable that both susceptible and non-susceptible people could be carrying vCJD, and transmit vCJD through the blood supply, but not be affected with vCJD themselves during their lifetime. Assuming this was the case then the upper limits on vCJD prevalence adopted in the analyses would be underestimates, and consequently the possible upper limits on annual numbers of blood donations from Australian donors carrying vCJD could be much larger than estimated at the time. It was also uncertain whether estimates of vCJD prevalence in UK residents applied uniformly across the whole UK resident population, or if they applied to Australian blood donors.

In addition to the assumptions in respect of the vCJD epidemiology there were also uncertainties in a number of other estimates used. These included; that the 1998 travel survey reflected the donor population in Australia in 2000; the proportion of blood donations excluded through donor deferral replaced by first time donors; accuracy of window period estimates for HIV and HCV NAT, and HBsAg; and the applicability to the 2000 period of the estimates of the median duration between donations in repeat donors infected with HIV, HCV and HBV during 1998. Further assumptions were that the prevalence of vCJD in Australian blood donors was proportional to duration of residence in the UK; and that donations made by infected HIV, HCV and HBV first time donors are made independently of infection point. It seemed reasonable to assume that the relative risk of exposure to BSE and hence risk of vCJD was proportional to the cumulative duration of residence in the UK during the risk years. There were, however, no data to assess whether the risk was directly proportional to duration of residence or not. Uncertainties in all the above estimates and assumptions indicated the need for caution when interpreting the modelling outcomes.

After careful consideration and with the support of the Australian Government the policy of deferring donations from donors who lived in the UK for a cumulative period of more than six months between 1980 and 1996 was instituted by the ARCBS commencing December 2000. This policy, which remains in place currently was heavily influenced by the analyses presented here which suggested that deferral of donors who lived in the UK during 1980 to 1996 may result in the removal of more donations from donors potentially infected with vCJD than would increase the number of donations infected with HIV, HCV or HBV made during the relevant window period.

Conceding the risk of evaluating decision making with the benefit of 'hindsight' it remains informative to retrospectively assess the accuracy of key policy decisions. With this aim in mind how does the 2000 ARCBS policy decision bear up in the face of current knowledge? On balance it appears quite favourable.

Perhaps the most important finding in support of the decision is that vCJD appears almost certainly to be transmissible from person to person by transfusion of labile components. At the time of writing four probable cases of transfusion transmitted vCJD (3 of which were symptomatic) have been identified in recipients of non leucodepleted red cell products [17,18]. In addition, the recent post-mortem discovery of abnormal prion protein in the spleen of an asymptomatic UK patient with haemophilia suggests, for the first time the possibility of vCJD transmission by fractionated plasma products [19]. This patient received several batches of UK sourced clotting factors including one batch manufactured from plasma from a donor who developed vCJD six months after donation. Since the patient also had several other possible routes of transmission including receiving red cell unit transfusions and undergoing several invasive biopsies, the finding does not conclusively establish plasma as a *bona fide* transmission route.

The transmissibility of vCJD by blood was at the time of the ARCBS policy decision suspected but hotly debated and therefore a key assumption in the risk assessment. Despite the risk being 'theoretical' rather than 'actual' at the time, it appears prudent to have applied the 'precautionary' approach of assuming transmissibility. In terms of the magnitude of the primary outbreak of vCJD in the UK the current total of 164 confirmed cases with a declining trend since 2000 indicates that initial modelling may have overestimated the prevalence and consequently the risk of vCJD in Australian donors. However, the level of asymptomatic infection and the potential for a secondary wave remains unclear. A retrospective UK study of vCJD infection in the UK using tonsil and appendix tissue found 3 positives of 12,674 samples [20]. This study indicates that the sub-clinical infection rate may be an order of magnitude higher than the observed reported case rate. A further larger UK study is pending which may clarify the asymptomatic carriage rate and potential for subsequent 'wave(s)' of infection. Modelling undertaken by investigators at the London School of Hygiene and Tropical Medicine and the National CJD Surveillance unit predicts that the potential for an epidemic of variant CJD via blood transfusion in the UK is possible but unlikely [21]. Using pessimistic modelling assumptions Clark and colleagues predicted that the size of the epidemic by 2080 was bounded above by 900 cases and that under optimistic assumptions where public health interventions were applied the upper boundary was reduced to 250 cases. The researchers concluded that although a self-sustaining epidemic was still possible the measures taken by the British Government and National Blood Service to protect transfusion recipients from contacting vCJD had been effective. In respect of the incidence of HIV, HCV and HBV infection in ARCBS donors it has shown a declining trend since the implementation of the policy indicating that the addition of new donors did not adversely impact the residual risk [22,23].

Despite the requirement to make a number of assumptions the risk modelling clearly added value to the decision making process in the case of the Australian vCJD donor deferral. Retrospectively these assumptions have generally held true and on balance the decision to implement the deferral has been justified by subsequent events.

Case study 2 – Implementing a Malaria Antibody Donor Screening Test for Potentially Exposed Blood Donors

Malaria is the leading cause of morbidity and mortality in the world having been responsible for more deaths than all other diseases and war combined. Malaria is caused by one of four species of human *Plasmodium*; *P. falciparum, P. vivax, P. ovale and P. malariae.* Transfusion Transmitted Malaria (TTM) was first reported in 1911 and remains today a rare but potentially serious complication of blood transfusion particularly when *P. falciparum* is the species involved [24]. Malaria parasites can survive for at least 3 weeks in refrigerated blood and although whole blood and red cell concentrates are most commonly implicated in TTM any component containing erythrocytes can potentially contain viable parasites. The incidence of TTM in non endemic countries ranges from 0 to 2 cases per million donations however may exceed 50 cases per million donations in countries were malaria is endemic [25,26]. The last reported case of TTM in Australia occurred in 1991 implying a residual risk not exceeding 1 in 10 million [27].

Until recently, and because of the lack of a reliable, high throughput screening test for malaria most blood services in non endemic countries have generally deferred donors with an identified malaria exposure risk. This strategy is sound from a risk management perspective evidenced by the low incidence of TTM. However the opportunity cost in terms of lost donors and donations is substantial and continually increasing as a result of the addition of new donor deferral criteria and the increasing propensity for international travel. For example the estimated loss of red blood cell donations associated with the ARCBS malaria donor deferral strategy in place in 2003 was 35,000 per annum [28].

In search of an alternative strategy to address this loss ARCBS embarked on a research project to identify potential candidate malaria tests sufficiently sensitive to maintain the existing level of residual risk for TTM. The latter constraint required the development of a novel risk model with the capability to estimate the change in residual risk for TTM associated with implementing a test based strategy [28]. The output from this model was pivotal in supporting a subsequent ARCBS policy decision to implement an antibody test based re-instatement strategy.

Model Development

The baseline for the model was the existing ARCBS donor deferral strategy which required donors to be categorised based on questioning as either ‘visitors’, ‘residents’ or ‘previously infected’ for malaria. Visitors were defined as donors who spent 6 months or less in a malaria endemic country. They were restricted to donating only plasma for fractionation for a period of 12 months after their return. Residents, defined as donors having spent a cumulative period of 6 months or more within the last 3 years in an endemic country, or donors with a previous history of malaria were restricted to donating only plasma for fractionation for a period of 3 years after their return to Australia, and for malarial history, absence of symptoms/cessation of therapy.

The proposed testing strategy involved implementing a test for malaria antibody for all donor categories above a minimum of 6 months after their return to Australia in the case of 'visitors' and 'residents', or after cessation of symptoms/therapy for 'previously infected' donors. The strategy involved collection and 'quarantine' of red cells pending a non reactive malaria antibody test (figure 1).

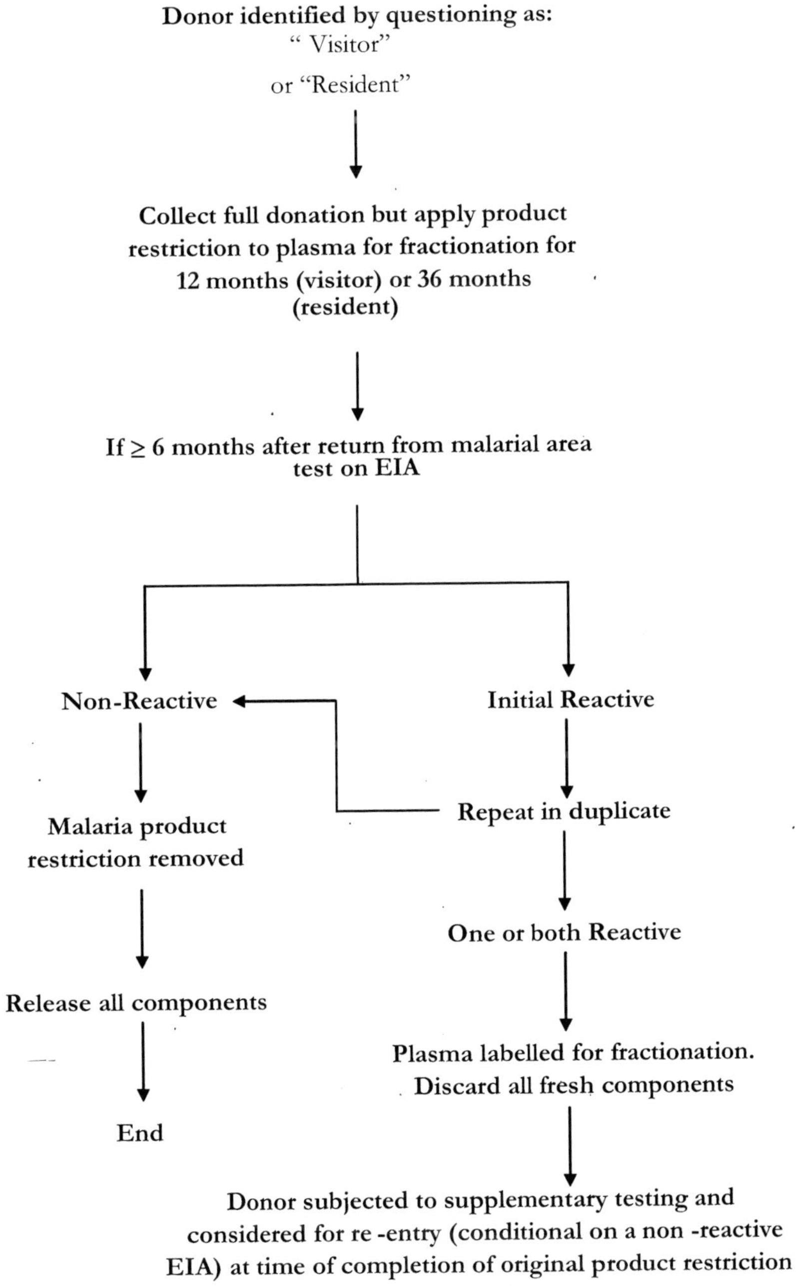

Figure 1. Malaria testing re-instatement protocol (Adapted with permission from reference 28).

In order to estimate the risk differential of implementing this testing strategy a mathematical model was developed which assumed that the risk differential was proportional to the probability that an infectious donor (i.e. parasitaemic) would successfully donate (i.e be asymptomatic at the time of donation) and subsequently test negative (i.e test false negative). It was determined that this probability could be sub-divided into three distinct components;

1. Incidence (I): The probability of an asymptomatic and parasitaemic donor donating more than 6 months after returning from an endemic area
2. Test Failure Rate (S): The probability that the donor in (1) above would also test 'non reactive'
3. Exposure risk: (E) the probability that the donor in (1) above was infected with a particular *Plasmodium* species

The following equation then represents the additional risk over existing (because none of these donations were issued for transfusion) of implementing the test based strategy.

$$\text{Risk} = (\text{I x S x E})$$

Method

Incidence

Because the incidence of parasitaemia in the sample of 375 ARCBS donors returned for more than 6 months was zero (i.e. none were determined to be parasitaemic) there was a requirement to indirectly estimate I. This estimate relied on the key assumption that the proportion of donors with parasitaemia who returned for 6 months or less versus more than 6 months would mirror the relative proportion of patients diagnosed within 6 months of initial infection compared to those diagnosed after 6 months. This proportion for *P. falciparum* and *P. vivax* (which represent the species most commonly associated with TTM in Australia) was derived using published data from three patient data sources including Western Australia (the donor population). In order to estimate I (incidence in donors returned for > 6 months) the proportion of diagnosed malaria was multiplied by the observed incidence in donors returned for less than 6 months (assumed to be at most 1/337 since none of 337 donors tested was parasitaemic) according to the following equation.

$$I^a = I^b \text{ x } (P1/P2)$$

Where;

I^a is the incidence of parasitaemia in donors returned (or asymptomatic and off treatment) for more than 6 months

I^b is the incidence of parasitaemia in donors returned (or asymptomatic and off treatment) for less than 6 months

P1 is the proportion of patients diagnosed within 6 months of infection

P2 is the proportion of patients diagnosed more than 6 months of infection

Test Failure Rate(S)

It was assumed that the test failure rate was dependent on the sensitivity of the test employed and could be represented by the following formula.

$$S = 1 - (\text{test sensitivity})$$

The best estimate of the test sensitivity would require an assessment of the ability of any candidate test to detect parasitaemia among blood donors eligible to be tested i.e. those where 6 months had elapsed since their last risk exposure. Due to the lack of a parasitaemic blood donor meeting these requirements in the ARCBS study such a direct assessment of test sensitivity was impossible. Consistent with the approach of other investigators test sensitivity was therefore assessed using confirmed positive parasitaemic samples from acutely infected patients diagnosed with clinical malaria.

Exposure risk

The probability of asymptomatic infection in a donor by individual *Plasmodium* species was derived by interrogating their travel histories. Each individual visit to a malarial risk country was assessed for risk per *Plasmodium* species by consulting the WHO 'International Travel and Health' website (www.who.int./ith). The risk per 'visit' was subdivided into 'low' or 'high' for each species and where more than one species was identified as a risk it was considered independently. (i.e. counted once against each species).

Results

The extrapolated incidence of asymptomatic parasitaemia (I) in donors eligible to be tested under the proposed strategy calculated as approximately 1 in 67,000 and 1 in 15,000 for *P. falciparum* and *P. vivax* respectively. Test sensitivity in acute clinical samples was estimated as 98.1(93.5-98.5%) for *P. falciparum* and 100(75.7-100%) for *P. vivax* although the latter was based only on 12 positive samples.

Applying this data to the risk model it was estimated that the additional risk of releasing an infected unit of blood in Australia associated with implementing the selected candidate assay (Newmarket malaria EIA) was approximately 1 in 6.1 (1.1- 34.6) million and 1 in 147,000 (26,000 – 833,000) donations tested for *P. falciparum* and *P. vivax* respectively. Assuming an average collection of 35,000 malaria risk donations per annum this translated to the release of one additional infected donation per 175 and 4.2 years for *P. falciparum* and *P. vivax* respectively.

Quantifying the TTM Risk Differential for Existing and Proposed Strategies

The estimated 'baseline' TTM risk in Australia of less than 1 in 10 million for the 2004 ARCBS deferral based strategy was derived by assessing the number of donations collected since the last documented case of TTM. Since this had occurred in 1991, and in the intervening period ARCBS had collected in excess of 10 million donations (ARCBS unpublished data) the risk estimate was less than 1 in 10 million (per donation collected). In order to derive a 'predicted' residual risk estimate for the proposed test based strategy this 'baseline' figure should be added to the risk increase derived from the modelling as follows;

Predicted risk post implementation	= baseline risk + additional risk
Baseline risk	=1 in 10 million [1x 10^{-7}] donations collected
Additional risk (*P falciparum*)	=1 in 175 million [6 x 10^{-9}] based on one additional *P. falciparum* infection per 175 years and an average annual collection of appromimately1 million donations
Predicted risk post implementation (*P. falciparum*)	= 1 x 10^{-7} + 6 x 10^{-9} = 1.06 x 10^{-9} or 1 in 9.4 million

Applying the same logic for *P. vivax* the risk of a TTM case involving this species calculated as approximately 1 in 3 million.

Risk/Benefit Analysis

In assessing the risk exposure associated with the change in strategy the quantitative data generated from the modelling was invaluable to ARCBS policy makers. However, this data needed to be interpreted within a full 'risk assessment framework' which considered all the relevant data and balanced the risks and benefits of the proposed policy change. Following are some considerations which underpinned the eventual ARCBS decision to implement a test based strategy;

1. Although any case of TTM can have serious consequences for the blood recipient the primary risk is associated with an undetected case of *P. falciparum* because fatalities with this species occur in approximately 10% of cases were it is the implicated organism [25]. In contrast, TTM cases involving the other three *Plasmodium* species rarely, if ever lead to a fatal outcome.

2. TTM cases cannot be avoided completely by deferring or restricting the donor to plasma for fractionation because asymptomatic carriage of parasites can persist for longer than the maximum three year period applied by ARCBS at the time. This is underscored by the existence of documented cases of asymptomatic carriage of parasites for as long as 53 years [29].

3. Errors in applying the deferral criteria correctly at the time of donation have lead to TTM cases. Mungai et al [25] found that 62% of donors implicated in a subsequent TTM case should have been deferred from donation had the existing exclusion criteria been correctly applied at the time.

4. Where donation restrictions apply (as in the ARCBS policy) errors in applying these can also lead the issue of potentially infectious components. Indeed the last case of TTM in Australia was an example of this. Despite eliciting correctly from the donor that they should have been restricted to plasma for fractionation based on a malarial risk exposure, red cells from the donor were issued for transfusion resulting in transmission of *P. falciparum* [27].

Chiodini et al highlighted the benefit of a dual strategy incorporating questioning and subsequent testing citing three TTM cases in the UK that would likely have been avoided [30].

5. Malaria antibody test based strategies had already been successfully implemented in Europe since the 1970's [31]. In particular French blood services had widely implemented a strategy for potentially exposed donors based on anti-malarial antibody detection by Indirect Immunofluorescence Antibody Test (IFAT). Donors returning from endemic countries were initially deferred for 4 months and subsequently tested between 4 months and three years after their return by IFAT. If IFAT negative they were considered malaria free and re-instated for donation of cellular components. The English National Blood Service had also implemented a similar strategy based on the same antibody EIA selected by ARCBS run in parallel with IFAT [32]. Donors were eligible to be tested after a minimum of period of 6 months had elapsed since their return from an endemic country and if negative re-instated for cellular component manufacture.

6. The predicted residual risk of TTM after implementation of the new strategy was similar to the existing risk of Transfusion Transmitted HIV (1 in 3.6 million) and less than the risk of Transfusion Transmitted HCV and HBV.

7. Based on the observed repeat reactive rate of the selected test (2.3%) it was predicted that over 17,000 additional RBC's would be made available for transfusion annually in Australia as a consequence of implementing the proposed strategy.

After balancing the risks against the significant predicted component savings the ARCBS, with the approval of the Australian regulator (Therapeutic Goods Administration-TGA) ratified the proposal to implement the proposed testing strategy with one minor revision. The minimum time before testing could be applied to eligible donors was revised downward from 6 to 4 months in line with the Council of Europe *Guide to the manufacture of blood and blood components* (11th Ed), the standard to which the ARCBS is required to comply.

Subsequent to approval of the Newmarket malaria EIA for use by the TGA the new policy commenced in July 2005. In terms of the outcome the results to date have been very favourable.(Manuscript submitted) At the time of writing and after 4 years testing the screening repeat reactive rate has remained stable at 2-3%. The recovery of RBC's has well exceeded predictions with the annual average exceeding 60,000 which represents almost 8% of RBC production. It is particularly pleasing that this has been achieved without any apparent increase in the residual risk. No new TTM cases were recorded and the observed TTM rate of zero since testing commenced was consistent with 95%CI predicted by the modelling providing empiric evidence for its accuracy.

CONCLUSION

Given the inevitable emergence of new infectious and non infectious threats necessitating further donor deferrals, Blood services will increasingly need to consider strategies to retain and make the most efficient use of their existing donor base. The two case studies presented in this chapter exemplify the value of risk modelling as a tool for evaluating and balancing the competing risks of blood safety and sufficiency. In the first case the modelling supports the application of a new deferral resulting in the loss of some 50,000 donations to protect blood recipients against a fatal disease. Counterbalancing this from a sufficiency standpoint, the second case study uses modelling to validate the application of a new testing strategy providing for early re-instatement of temporarily deferred donors consequently recovering more than 60,000 additional red blood cell donations per annum. Importantly, although not inter-related the net impact of implementing both strategies is a virtual 'status quo' in terms of sufficiency and safety.

References

[1] Weinburg P, Hounshell J, Sherman LA, Godwin J, Ali S, Tomori C, Bennet CL. Legal, financial, and public health consequences of HIV contamination of blood and blood products in the 1980's and 1990's. *Ann Intern Med.* 2002;136:312-9.

[2] Starr D. *Blood: An epic history of medicine and commerce*. New York: Alfred A. Knoph 1999.

[3] Hergon E, Moutel G, Duchange N, Bellier L, Rouger P, Herve C. Risk management in transfusion after the HIV blood contamination crisis in France: the impact of the precautionary principle. *Transfus Med Rev*. 2005 Oct;19(4):273-80.

[4] European Environment Agency. http.//glossary.eea.eu.International/EEAGlossary/P/precautionary_principle. 1992.

[5] Moreno JD. "Creeping precautionism" and the blood supply. *Transfusion*. 2003 Jul;43(7):840-2.

[6] Brown P, Rohwer RG, Dunstan BC, MacAuley C, Gajdusek DC, Drohan WN. The distribution of infectivity in blood components and plasma derivatives in experimental models of transmissible spongiform encephalopathy. *Transfusion*. 1998 Sep;38(9):810-6.

[7] Farrugia A. The regulatory pendulum in transfusion medicine. *Transfus Med Rev*. 2002 Oct;16(4):273-82.

[8] Houston F, Foster JD, Chong A, Hunter N, Bostock CJ. Transmission of BSE by blood transfusion in sheep. *Lancet*. 2000 Sep 16;356(9234):999-1000.

[9] Det Norske Veritas. Risk of infection from variant CJD in blood. http://wwwdnvcouk/Binaries/vCJD_Update_Report_tc27-74414pdf. 2004.

[10] Hewitt PE, Llewelyn CA, Mackenzie J, Will RG. Creutzfeldt-Jakob disease and blood transfusion: results of the UK Transfusion Medicine Epidemiological Review study. *Vox Sang*. 2006 Oct;91(3):221-30.

[11] Correll PK, Law MG, Seed CR, Gust A, Buring M, Dax EM, Keller AJ, Kaldor JM. Variant Creutzfeldt-Jakob disease in Australian blood donors: estimation of risk and the impact of deferral strategies. *Vox Sang*. 2001 Jul;81(1):6-11.

[12] Ghani AC, Ferguson NM, Donnelly CA, Anderson RM. Predicted vCJD mortality in Great Britain. *Nature*. 2000 Aug 10;406(6796):583-4.

[13] Ironside JW, Hilton DA, Ghani A, Johnston NJ, Conyers L, McCardle LM, Best D. Retrospective study of prion-protein accumulation in tonsil and appendix tissues. *Lancet*. 2000 May 13;355(9216):1693-4.

[14]Kleinman S, Busch MP, Korelitz JJ, Schreiber GB. The incidence/window period model and its use to assess the risk of transfusion-transmitted human immunodeficiency virus and hepatitis C virus infection. *Transfus Med Rev.* 1997 Jul;11(3):155-72.

[15]Muller-Breitkreutz K. Results of viral marker screening of unpaid blood donations and probability of window period donations in 1997. EPFA Working Group on Quality Assurance. *Vox Sang.* 2000;78(3):149-57.

[16]Mimms LT, Mosley JW, Hollinger FB, Aach RD, Stevens CE, Cunningham M, Vallari DV, Barbosa LH, Nemo GJ. Effect of concurrent acute infection with hepatitis C virus on acute hepatitis B virus infection. *BMJ.* 1993 Oct 30;307(6912):1095-7.

[17]Hewitt PE, Llewelyn CA, Mackenzie J, Will RG. Three reported cases of variant Creutzfeldt-Jakob disease transmission following transfusion of labile blood components. *Vox Sang.* 2006 Nov;91(4):348.

[18]Health Protection Agency. Fourth case of transfusion-associated variant-CJD infection. *Health Protection Report* 2007. 2007;1(3).

[19]Heallth Protection Agency. vCJD abnormal prion protein found in a patient with haemophilia at post mortem. available at www.hpa.org.uk 2009.

[20]Hilton DA, Ghani AC, Conyers L, Edwards P, McCardle L, Ritchie D, Penney M, Hegazy D, Ironside JW. Prevalence of lymphoreticular prion protein accumulation in UK tissue samples. *J Pathol.* 2004 Jul;203(3):733-9.

[21]Clarke P, Will RG, Ghani A. Is there the potential for an epidemic of variant Creutzfeldt-Jacob disease via blood transfusion in the UK? *J R Soc Interface.* 2007;4(15):675-84.

[22]Seed CR, Cheng A, Ismay SL, Bolton WV, Kiely P, Cobain TJ, Keller AJ. Assessing the accuracy of three viral risk models in predicting the outcome of implementing HIV and HCV NAT donor screening in Australia and the implications for future HBV NAT. *Transfusion.* 2002 Oct;42(10):1365-72.

[23]Seed CR, Kiely P, Keller AJ. Residual risk of transfusion transmitted human immunodeficiency virus, hepatitis B virus, hepatitis C virus and human T lymphotrophic virus. *Intern Med J.* 2005 Oct;35(10):592-8.

[24]Katz LM. Transfusion induced malaria. In: Brecher ME, ed. *Bacterial and Parasitic contamination of blood products. Bethesda* 2003:127-51.

[25]Mungai M, Tegtmeier G, Chamberland M, Parise M. Transfusion-transmitted malaria in the United States from 1963 through 1999. *N Engl J Med.* 2001 Jun 28;344(26):1973-8.

[26]Bruce-Chwatt LJ. Transfusion malaria revisited. *Trop Dis Bull.* 1982 Oct;79(10):827-40.

[27]Whyte GS. Therepeutic goods and malaria. *Medical Journal of Australia.* 1992;157:439-40.

[28]Seed CR, Cheng A, Davis TM, Bolton WV, Keller AJ, Kitchen A, Cobain TJ. The efficacy of a malarial antibody enzyme immunoassay for establishing the reinstatement status of blood donors potentially exposed to malaria. *Vox Sang.* 2005 Feb;88(2):98-106.

[29]Besson P, Robert JF, Reviron J, Richard-Lenoble D, Gentilini M. [2 cases of transfusional malaria. Attempted prevention combining an indirect immunofluorescence test with clinical selection critera]. *Rev Fr Transfus Immunohematol.* 1976 Jun;19(2):369-73.

[30]Chiodini PL, Hartley S, Hewitt PE, Barbara JA, Lalloo K, Bligh J, Voller A. Evaluation of a malaria antibody ELISA and its value in reducing potential wastage of red cell donations from blood donors exposed to malaria, with a note on a case of transfusion-transmitted malaria. *Vox Sang.* 1997;73(3):143-8.

[31]Silvie O, Thellier M, Rosenheim M, Datry A, Lavigne P, Danis M, Mazier D. Potential value of Plasmodium falciparum-associated antigen and antibody detection for screening of blood donors to prevent transfusion-transmitted malaria. *Transfusion*. 2002 Mar;42(3):357-62.

[32]Kitchen AD, Lowe PH, Lalloo K, Chiodini PL. Evaluation of a malarial antibody assay for use in the screening of blood and tissue products for clinical use. *Vox Sang*. 2004 Oct;87(3):150-5.

In: Transfusion - Think About It
Editor: Trevor J. Cobain

ISBN 978-1-61668-969-8

Chapter 11

INFECTIOUS DISEASE THREATS TO THE BLOOD SUPPLY

Anthony Keller
Australian Red Cross Blood Service, Perth, Western Australia.

ABSTRACT

Having made very significant progress in minimizing the risk of transmission of HIV, Hepatitis C and Hepatitis B by blood transfusion, new risks of infectious disease transmission continually emerge. Thus new infections and mutated virulent strains of existing agents emerge with potential or actual risks to blood safety [1,2]. Furthermore the geographic ranges and prevalence rates of well-known infectious agents are expanding. These phenomena are collectively termed emerging or re-emerging infections and are the subject of continuing research particularly by the transfusion community [3,4].

INTRODUCTION

This chapter addresses firstly those well known transfusion transmissible infections for which sensitive and specific screening tests have reduced the risk of transmission to negligible levels. Secondly, a number of emerging and re-emerging viral infections directly relevant to the safety of the blood supply in Australia (but which also impact other countries), are examined.

Thirdly the chapter describes general risk assessment principles using examples of infectious agents that are considered to be a potential problem for the Australian blood supply but have not yet been associated with transfusion transmission

Transmission by Transfusion

A number of infectious agents are known to be transmissible by blood transfusion and vigorous effort goes into preventing or minimising such transmission. Classically, blood services have been concerned with a number of transfusion-transmitted viruses (TTV) that exhibit the following characteristics:

1) Cause mild or asymptomatic infections such that infected potential donors would present (and be accepted) for donation (e.g. Hepatitis A)
2) Have clinical latency (incubation) periods of years to decades (e.g. hepatitis B and C (HBV, HCV), human immunodeficiency virus (HIV), human T-cell lymphotropic virus (HTLV))
3) Might cause a 'carrier' state of infection (e.g. HIV, HBV and HCV)
4) Might cause a 'latent' state of infection in host cells by incorporating their own DNA in the host's DNA (e.g. HIV,HTLV and cytomegalovirus (CMV))
5) Would be present in blood components (e.g. HIV either in plasma as RNA or as proviral DNA in leukocytes)
6) Would be stable under the conditions at which blood components are stored.

Historically, most infections transmissible by transfusion have been characterised by a prolonged, silent carrier state with the infectious agent circulating in the blood but not causing symptoms. However, some infections with very short period of infectivity in the blood (i.e., a few days) have been transmitted via transfusion [5]. Indeed, Kleinman highlights that, "WNV represents a prototype of a class of pathogens not previously recognised as a transfusion threat" [6]. These pathogens cause acute, short-term viraemia in asymptomatic potential blood donors with consequent rapid spread via localised epidemics which are temporally and geographically restricted. The transmission of WNV by blood transfusion in North America highlighted the potential of other arboviruses, e.g. dengue, to pose a similar threat to blood safety. Nonetheless, the overall picture is that the main risk of transfusion-transmitted infections (TTI) arises from persistent infections. Because of this persistence, the presence of detectable antibody to the agent generally indicates the likelihood of continuing infection (and infectivity by transfusion), rather than clearance of the virus.

With some exceptions (e.g. Hepatitis B) the detection of antibodies to infectious agents has formed the basis for the classical serological approaches to the routine testing of donated blood for TTV. In Australia for example, all blood donations are routinely screened for the following viruses: HIV-1 and 2, Hepatitis B and C, and HTLV-I and II [7]. Selected donations are also screened for CMV antibodies to provide CMV seronegative blood components for transfusion to immuno-compromised patients at risk of severe and occasionally life-threatening complications. In addition, some blood services internationally screen for other transfusion transmitted viruses including human Erythrovirus (formerly Parvo B19), Hepatitis A virus and West Nile virus (WNV) [8].

The cornerstones of prevention of transfusion transmitted infections are epidemiological surveillance, rigorous donor selection using a comprehensive questionnaire and interview to exclude donors at high-risk. The application of increasingly sensitive screening tests and pathogen inactivation for plasma derived products are also essential. These strategies have substantially reduced the risk of transmission of HIV, HBV, HCV and HTLV in Australia [9].

Nucleic Acid Testing (NAT) for HCV and HIV-1 RNA, implemented in 2000 in Australia has further reduced the risk of transmission of these viruses by transfusion [10]. Risk modelling conducted by the ARCBS subsequent to the implementation of NAT estimated the residual risk (i.e. the probability of releasing an infectious unit) for these viruses to be extremely low, ranging from approximately1 in 1 million (HBV) to 1 in 7.6 million (HIV) [7]. This confirms that Australia has one of the safest blood supplies in the world in terms of these pathogens. However, as the rapid emergence of WNV in North America has demonstrated, there is no room for complacency.

Emerging and Re-emerging Infections

The response to WNV however demonstrates the power of technology to mitigate the risk of potential viral threats. The USA and Canadian Blood Services responded to the threat of WNV demonstrating that the rapidity with which molecular-based screening tests can be introduced is truly startling [11].

Notably, the major risk to the blood supply from a significant new viral disease outbreak may not be from TTI but rather the effect it would have on the maintenance of adequate staffing levels and eligible blood donors. An example might be the emergence of pandemic influenza strain that could severely compromise the ability to maintain an adequate blood supply [12]. To mitigate this in Australia the ARCBS has commenced dialogue with the relevant Australian Government agencies to develop a comprehensive response plan. Some priorities of this plan include: the continued protection of the health and wellbeing of staff and donors, enhanced infection control measures for blood collection facilities and modifications to donor selection criteria to boost eligible donors. The ARCBS has also engaged with international Blood Services through the Alliance of Blood Operators (ABO) to develop and share relevant pandemic planning information.

By definition, a truly emerging infectious agent would be one that has newly entered a population and is not simply an established agent that has been detected for the first time. An agent can emerge either de novo by mutation or by crossing a species barrier to enter the human disease chain. HIV is an example of a truly emergent infectious agent. The distinction between emerging infectious agents and emerging problems was emphasised by Alter [13]. For example, pre-existing bacteria emerged as problems when the frequency of platelet transfusions increased and when room temperature storage conditions for optimal platelet survival created a fertile environment for bacterial growth. The rapid spread of West Nile Virus [WNV] across North America is an example of a re-emerging agent. It is an organism that has caused outbreaks in Africa, the Middle East and Southern Europe in the past and represented a minimal transfusion risk. This changed rapidly when it was imported into the USA where there was a suitable vector and a susceptible animal and human population. The increased virulence of the virus has also been implicated in its rapid spread across North America.

Australian Arboviruses-Examples of Emerging Threats to the Blood Supply

Arboviruses or arthropod-born viruses are vector-borne viruses that have been associated with human disease in Australia. These viruses are transmitted between blood-feeding arthropod vectors (mosquitoes in the Australian region) and susceptible vertebrate hosts and undergo a replicative cycle in both. The viraemia in the host usually only lasts for a few days or weeks, after which the host normally develops life-long immunity to the virus [14].

Over 65 arboviruses have been reported from countries in the Australasian geographic region, but only a few have been implicated in human disease and only one (dengue virus) where transfusion transmission has been reported [14,15,16]. Six of the viruses are of particular concern and their characteristics and potential for transfusion transmission are summarised in Table 1.

Table 1. Arboviral Disease Notification data for 2007 compared with their five year average rates [35]

Virus	Number of Notifications		Notification Rates per 100,000	
	2007	Last 5 Years (Mean)	2007	Last 5 Years (Mean)
Barmah Forest Virus	1,695	1,366	8.1	6.7
Dengue Flavivirus	318	358	1.5	1.8
Flavivirus (NEC)*	23	51	0.1	0.3
Japanese Encephalitis	0	1	0	0
Kunjin	0	9	0	0
Murray Valley encephalitis	0	2	0	0
Ross River Virus	4,143	3,513	19.7	17.3

* Not elsewhere classified.

Ross River virus [RRV] belongs to the alphavirus genus. Each year it causes hundreds of cases of a debilitating and frequently persistent disease known as epidemic polyarthritis throughout Australasia. Barmah Forest virus (BFV), another alphavirus, causes a similar disease to RRV and has recently emerged as an increasing cause of human disease on mainland Australia [14].

The genus, flavivirus includes Murray Valley encephalitis virus [MVEV] and Kunjin virus [KUNV] that are the aetiological agents of rare but potentially lethal encephalitic diseases known as Australian encephalitis, and Kunjin encephalitis, respectively [14].

Another flavivirus of the JE sero-group is West Nile virus(WNV). Phylogenetically, it is closely related to the Australian KUNV. Until recently, WNV was endemic in a large part of Africa, Southern and South-eastern Europe, the Middle East, and the Western part of the Indian subcontinent where it periodically resulted in large, but generally geographically restricted, outbreaks. In those areas, it would not qualify as an emerging infection. However, in 1999, an outbreak of WNV infection occurred in New York City with 66 human cases and 22 deaths [17]. By 2002, the disease had spread to most US states and into Canada, with 4,156 human cases and 284 deaths that year. Notably, the number of reported cases would have significantly underestimated the true infection rate since; a) reporting of symptomatic cases was likely incomplete, and b) most infections are asymptomatic. By the end of 2002, more than 60 suspected transfusion transmitted cases of WNV had been reported and 23 of these were confirmed. Changes to donor screening programs were rapidly introduced and by July 2003, nucleic acid testing (NAT) for routine screening of blood donations in small pools was in place throughout the US and Canada. At the peak of the epidemic, the estimated population infection rate in some US states (inferred retrospectively from the incidence of WNV NAT positive donations) was as high as 3/1,000 [18]. Transfusion transmission of WNV is rare to absent outside North America and Australian virologists have speculated that KUNV exposure would offer some degree of protection in Australia [19]. However, it is not inconceivable that a problem could occur with KUNV and/or MVEV in Australasia. Dengue Flavivirus (DENV), particularly serotypes 1-4, are the most important arboviruses of humans, infecting 30-70 million individuals annually in tropical and subtropical regions, including Australasia [20]. Most DENV infections lead to dengue fever, a self limiting febrile disease, but in some cases patients develop severe dengue hemorrhagic fever or dengue shock syndrome (DHF/DSS). DENV infections are probably not endemic in Australia but have caused increasingly frequent outbreaks in north-eastern Australia following re-introduction of the viruses in viraemic travellers. The first outbreak of Japanese encephalitis virus (JEV) in Australia occurred in the Torres Strait of northern Australia in early 1995. This flavivirus causes more than 50,000 clinical cases annually in eastern and southern Asia, with a 25% case-fatality rate. Recent serosurveys indicate that JEV may also be regularly active in PNG. The geographic range of JEV has increased significantly over the last three or four decades [14].

Other arboviruses such as the alphavirus, Sindbis, the flaviviruses, Alfuy, Edge Hill, Kokobera and Stratford and the bunyaviruses, Gan Gan and Trubanaman are not discussed as they appear to cause only mild symptoms and have not been implicated in transfusion transmission and are therefore of less concern although they are all found in Australia [20].

Other Viruses

The alphavirus, Chikungunya (CHIKV) is responsible for widespread epidemics, most recently in Mauritius and Reunion Island, the Seychelles and India. Chikungunya causes an arthralgic disease which until recently was not associated with severe morbidity or mortality. Recent outbreaks have demonstrated a potential for symptoms to range from mild to severe, with 237 deaths implicated among some 265,000 clinical cases in the 2006 Reunion outbreak [22]. To date there have been no documented Australian cases of autochthonous Chikungunya infection, but there is an increasing number of imported cases [23,24]. An unprecedented localised CHIKV outbreak in Northern Italy during 2007 well illustrates the potential for rapid spread of infectious disease agents. The establishment of the CHIKV mosquito vector *Aedes albopictus* in the region and the subsequent importation of CHIKV via an infected traveller established a local epidemic leading to the precautionary discontinuation of blood collection [25]. Unlike WNV which is proven to be 'transfusion transmitted', to date there have been no reported cases of transfusion transmission associated with Chikungunya. However, a cautionary approach is indicated given that, like DENV transfusion transmission may not be immediately evident during large epidemics where mosquito borne transmission predominates.

Viral Haemorrhagic Fevers (VHF) are a group of highly infectious and usually fatal diseases caused by several different viruses. Four VHF [Ebola, Marburg, Crimean-Congo Lassa and the recently described Arenavirus] are quarantinable diseases in Australia. The viruses are transmitted between humans through body fluids and airborne droplets. They are not considered a major transfusion risk in Australia because of their rarity and the rapidity with which symptoms develop and the high mortality rate. However, serological evidence of asymptomatic infection has been reported with Ebola [26], so transmission by blood transfusion could potentially occur.

Two relatively recent members of the paramyxovirus group of viruses, Hendra and Nipah, have been transmitted to humans via horses and pigs, respectively. Four people in Australia, have been infected by Hendra virus and two died [27]. A Nipah virus outbreak in Malaysia in 1999, was characterised by severe fever, malaise and encephalopathy and killed 30% of 270 people. While no human-to human transmission was observed actions have been taken during outbreaks to protect the Australian blood supply [28]. A novel Arenavirus isolated from a single donor who subsequently died of a brain haemorrhage was transmitted to three organ transplant recipients in Victoria in early 2007 (all three of whom died) [29]. This previously unknown virus appears to be related to lymphocytic choriomeningitis virus (LCMV), a member of the genus Arenavirus of the Arenaviridae family of the bipartite genome RNA viruses. More recently yet another as yet unnamed Arenavirus isolated from a Zambian patient in South Africa lead to four fatalities. (Global Alert and Response, World Health Organisation, 10 October 2008). Rodents are the reservoir hosts of almost all Arenaviruses and, accordingly, LCMV infection in humans may occur in regions of high rodent density. Although transplantation transmission of this distinct, as well as prototype LCMV appears to be well established, it is unclear whether these viruses are 'passengers' or directly responsible for tissue-rejection illness and death. Although transfusion transmission has not been implicated to date, the close correlation between organ and blood transmission of many other viruses (e.g. WNV, HIV, HCV) is reason for due concern.

There is evidence that the highly contagious Severe Acute Respiratory Syndrome [SARS] virus, which emerged in November 2002, did have a viraemic phase, at least during symptomatic disease [5]. However, there is no evidence (from past studies, checking donors/donations against SARS patient registries and surveillance of blood donor populations for SARS antibody) that SARS was transmissible by blood transfusion. Nevertheless, the WHO has made recommendations for blood deferral in relation to SARS and in Australia, the ARCBS donor screening questionnaire includes questions that should identify (symptomatic) donors. Specific geographical deferrals were introduced during the SARS outbreak. There is evidence that the highly lethal H5N1 avian influenza virus that has spread globally since 2003 has a short viraemic phase while symptoms are present. Transmissibility studies are underway in the US but the risk of asymptomatic H5N1 viraemia or infection with other influenza viruses novel to humans remains unknown [30]. Finally, three novel viruses were identified as a result of molecular viral discovery programs searching for the agents responsible for unexplained cases of hepatitis. HGV (hepatitis G virus, or GB virus type C), TT-virus and SEN virus have all subsequently demonstrated the ability to be transmitted by blood products and their prevalence in various populations ranges from1.8 to 36% [31,32]. Initially all three were proposed as possible agents non A-E hepatitis. Comprehensive clinical studies have so far failed to demonstrate that any of these agents cause human hepatitis and they are considered to be 'agents searching for a disease' [33]. Accordingly, no specific measures to protect the blood supply from these agents have been implemented.

SURVEILLANCE

Surveillance is fundamental to the prevention and control of communicable diseases. In Australia human cases of arbovirus infection are monitored through the National Notifiable Diseases Surveillance System (NNDSS) [34]. States and Territories each maintain separate jurisdictional surveillance, but they all report their results, using common case definitions, to the Commonwealth Department of Health and Ageing.

The viral diseases monitored are those caused by RRV, MVEV and KUNV, DENV (all serotypes) and JEV. Table 1 shows disease notification data for 2007 compared with their five-year average rates are extracted from the NNDSS.

Again, it should be noted that the number of reported cases would have significantly underestimated the true infection rate since reporting of symptomatic cases was certainly incomplete. Notifications for each disease are also regularly analysed and reported in the Department's quarterly, *Communicable Diseases Intelligence* [35]. More up-to-date statistics are available from the Communicable Diseases Australia website [35]. Complementing these data, fortnightly teleconferences by state and territory epidemiologists with their national counterparts allow recent and local disease outbreaks to be discussed and monitored. Flavivirus sero-conversion is detected in sentinel chicken flocks in four Australian States/Territories. Flocks in Western Australia (30 flocks), Victoria (10), New South Wales (7) and the Northern Territory (9) are used to provide an early warning of increased levels of MVEV and KUNV activity in the region. During the 2003/04 season, low levels of flavivirus activity were detected in Northern Australia with both MVEV and KUNV virus activity detected in the Kimberley and Pilbara regions of Western Australia and in the Northern Territory. These programs are funded by the state health departments. Flocks are sampled regularly for antibody testing with a sensitive enzyme immunoassay. Each state has a contingency plan in the event of an outbreak. Australia also maintains a sentinel pig program for JEV, with pig herds in northern Queensland, the Northern Territory and the Torres Strait Islands (TSI). In addition to the TSI outbreak detected in 1995 (and in most years since), an outbreak was also detected on mainland Australia in 1998 [28]. In 2005, there were two cases of MVEV infection reported, the first in a 30-year-old male from Normanton Queensland, and the second in a 3-year-old boy from a NT community who was treated at Royal Darwin Hospital. The latter displayed mild illness and completely recovered. His community was located near an extensive freshwater wetland with numerous water birds and frequent high numbers of common banded mosquitoes *Culex annulirostris* and *Culex palpalis*: two vectors of MVEV [29]. Arbovirus transmission cycles are complex and poorly understood in Australasia, particularly with regard to the role of the environment.

Thus, the public health response to the threat of increased activity of these viruses must include further research into the ecologies of these viruses, their known and potential vectors and hosts and environmental conditions that predispose to outbreaks. ARCBS monitors changes in epidemiological infectious disease patterns through national and international networks and publications so that it can proactively move to protect the blood supply when emergent or re-emergent infectious agents threaten the safety of the blood supply.

Climate

Changes in climatic conditions may significantly alter the ecology and epidemiology of arboviruses and thus their potential to cause outbreaks of human disease [14]. Expected climatic changes resulting from the 'greenhouse effect', such as increased rainfall with subsequent flooding and rising sea levels (with greater tidal penetration of coastlines), are likely to enhance breeding of mosquito vectors. In Australia for example major outbreaks of RRV disease have been linked to extreme rainfall events and short term rises in sea level. MVEV activity has also been associated with heavy rainfall and flooding. Increases in temperature may accelerate vector life cycles and shorten extrinsic incubation of arboviruses. This would mean vectors would become infectious more quickly. These conditions expected to lead to higher levels of virus activity and greater exposure of humans to the viruses. Therefore, surveillance for further spread of other dangerous arboviruses such as JEV and DENV is imperative.

Infectious Diseases Emerging Viral Threats

Apart from climate change, there are also other reasons why viral pathogens might expand their geographical distribution, such as increased international travel, increased international animal and bird movement, and deforestation.

Interventions

The risk of transfusion from emerging infections needs to be managed systematically. In general, a systematic approach should include a broad mechanism of surveillance to identify emerging infections, followed by a process to assess whether the agent could be transmitted by transfusion.

Increasingly expensive interventions to reduce microbial risks which have been of may need to be applied are: 1) education and selection of voluntary donors; 2) sensitive and specific serological and/or Nucleic Acid testing ; 3) leucodepletion of all blood components (implementation of Universal Leucodepletion of red cells and platelets was completed in Australia in October 2008) ; 4) viral inactivation of fractionated products and, as a possible option for the future; 5) pathogen reduction for fresh blood components; 6) introduction of 'blood substitutes'; 7) vaccination of donors and 8) blood conservation strategies to minimize inappropriate transfusion [3,36].

Currently available interventions include: measures based on selection of epidemiologically safe populations from which donors are drawn; measures based on a history elicited from the donor, leading to permanent or temporary deferral; and test methods designed to detect evidence of infection or infectivity with the agent in question. These measures need to be constantly reviewed as the strain on maintaining, managing and financing the blood supply increases.

A recent ARCBS report affirms the effectiveness of stringent donor selection criteria in reducing the risk of TTI. In the report, the prevalence of HIV, HCV, HBV and HTLV in accepted blood donors was 50-350 times less than in the Australian population [9]. In the absence of validated screening tests targeted donor questioning can also be an effective measure to minimise the TTI risk. A good example of this is the use of geographically based exclusion of donors during seasonal dengue outbreaks in Northern Australia [37]. Subsequent to a declared dengue outbreak, all ARCBS donors are questioned and if they have travelled to the affected area they are temporarily disallowed from donating fresh blood components (although they may donate plasma for further manufacture that includes highly effective viral inactivation procedures). Once the epidemic is declared over, donor restrictions are lifted and dengue specific questioning is curtailed.

Transfusion-Transmitted vCJD and its Consequences

The epidemic of bovine spongiform encephalopathy (BSE) in cattle in the United Kingdom, that began in 1980 and the subsequent outbreak of variant Creutzfeldt-Jakob Disease (vCJD) in humans that began in 1996 heralded a new fear for the safety of the blood supply, not only in the UK but throughout the world [38,39].

The disease, which had originally appeared in cattle, is caused by a prion (a misfolded protein). The normal protein PrP^{C}, a membrane sialoglycoprotein, converts from an alpha helical conformation to a beta sheet structure (PrP^{SC} or PrP^{TSE}), forming abnormal aggregates resistant to protease digestion. Prion propagation probably occurs through template-induced conversion of further PrP^{C} to PrP^{TSE}. The aggregates of PrP^{TSE} accumulate in the central nervous system, and these aggregates and associated abnormal cellular functions cause irreversible brain damage [40].

Fears that the disease might be transmissible by transfusion were confirmed by early studies in rodent animal models [41]. Sheep experimentally infected with BSE and scrapie, a transmissible prion encephalopathy in sheep, confirmed transmission by whole blood and buffy coat [42]. In a longitudinal study of transmission of prions by transfusion in sheep, the reported transmission rates were 36% for BSE and 43% for scrapie [43]. Three of the eight affected transfusion recipient sheep were alive for up to 7 years without showing signs of clinical disease. The majority of transmissions resulted from blood collected from donors at greater than 50% of the estimated incubation period. The authors concluded that infectivity titres in blood were substantial and/or that blood transfusion is a particularly efficient means of transmission.

The epidemic of vCJD in humans beginning in 1996 was caused by the ingestion of abnormal BSE prions in beef. The disease is a progressive encephalopathy manifested by spongioform degeneration of the brain with florid amyloid plaques and neuronal loss. Early symptoms are neuropsychiatric and include anxiety, depression, dysaesthesia and ataxia. Patients develop progressive dementia, myoclonus and choreoathetosis with an average clinical course to death of 6 months to 2 years (median 14 months).

The disease predominantly affects young adults and is invariably fatal. The first cases of vCJD occurred in the UK in 1996. To date there have been a total of 211 cases in humans, with the majority occurring in the United Kingdom (168 cases) and France (25 cases), several cases in other European countries and one case in Saudi Arabia [44]. The USA has reported three cases and Canada one case, but Japan is the only country in Asia to have reported a case to date – these cases appear to be related to residence in the United Kingdom during the risk years (Table 2).

Table 2. vCJD Cases Worldwide

Country	Total Number of Primary Cases	Total Number of Secondary Cases: Blood Transfusion	Cumulative Residence in UK >6 Months During Period 1980-1996
UK	165	3	168
France	25	-	1
Republic of Ireland	4	-	2
Italy	1	-	0
USA	3†	-	2
Canada	1	-	1
Saudi Arabia	1	-	0
Japan	1*	-	0
Netherlands	3	-	0
Portugal	2	-	0
Spain	5	-	0

† the third US patient with vCJD was born and raised in Saudi Arabia and has lived permanently in the United States since late 2005. According to the US case-report, the patient was most likely infected as a child when living in Saudi Arabia.

* the case from Japan had resided in the UK for 24 days in the period 1980-1996.

Ref: Adapted from table at http://www.eurocjd.ed.ac.uk/vcjdworldeuro.htm

All confirmed clinical cases to date have been homozygous for methionine at codon 129 of the PRNP gene.

The first putative transfusion transmitted case in humans occurred in the UK in 2004. The risks of prion transmission associated with transfusion have been extensively reviewed by Lefrère and Hewitt [45]. Four cases associated with transfusion of fresh components, namely non-leucodepleted red cells, have now been reported although one of the cases was subclinical with vCJD detected in lymphoreticular tissues at post mortem. None of the cases in France have been associated with transfusion, even though three of the reported cases had donated blood [46].

This year, UK Health authorities reported a patient with haemophilia who showed pathological signs of abnormal prion protein (vCJD) in the spleen after dying of unrelated causes. Although he had received 14 units of red cells, none of the donors had gone on to develop vCJD. A risk analysis showed that there is a 99 percent probability of the infection being caused by clotting concentrates [47].

Although the number of vCJD cases in the United Kingdom has decreased since 2000, the number of asymptomatic subclinical or preclinical cases is essentially unknown. In the absence of a specific and sensitive screening test it is impossible to know the extent of the disease in its subclinical or preclinical form. One retrospective study of 14,674 tonsillectomy and appendicectomy specimens in 2004 revealed that three appendicectomy specimens were positive for vCJD with an estimated prevalence of 237 carriers per million population [48]. Although all clinical cases of vCJD described to date have been methionine/ methionine (M/M) homozygous at the PRNP codon 129 of the PrP^{C} gene it is noteworthy that two of the three asymptomatic appendicectomy cases were valine/valine (V/V) homozygous at codon 129. Furthermore, while the three clinical transfusion transmitted cases were M/M homozygous, the fourth subclinical case was methionine/valine (M/V) heterozygous at codon 129 [49].

A more recent cross sectional opportunistic survey of anonymous tonsil specimens in Britain, examined 63,007 samples using two enzyme immunoassays [50]. None of the samples tested were unequivocally reactive in both assays. The authors concluded that the observed prevalence of PrP^{CJD} in tonsils in the 1961-95 birth cohort (when the risk of exposure to bovine spongiform encephalopathy was high) was 0/32,661 (95% confidence interval 0-113 per million). In the subset 1961-85 birth cohort the prevalence was still zero (95% confidence interval of 0-289 per million which was consistent with the previous survey). Two further studies may provide further information about prevalence, a large scale survey of appendices due to commence this year and a suggested study of post-mortem spleen samples in an older population.

The declining number of cases of vCJD since 2000 has not led to confidence that the outbreak is over. On the contrary there is concern that a second wave may occur in the future in heterozygous methionine/valine (M/V) individuals (50% of the population) and in valine/valine (V/V) homozygotes (11% of the population). This is supported not only by the heterozygous patient who died from a non-vCJD related disease five years after receiving the contaminated red cell transfusion and the two asymptomatic valine homozygous patients identified as positive for the prion protein, but also by the recently reported suspected vCJD heterozygous patient in the UK [49,50,51]. One possibility is that while it is possible that individuals heterozygous for methionine and valine or homozygous for valine at codon 129 of the PRNP gene may remain asymptomatic, they may act as sources of infection for others. Thus, as subclinical carriers such individuals could act as sources of infection either via contaminated surgical instruments or through blood transfusion for other persons homozygous for methionine at codon 129.

On the other hand, using a simulation approach the number of future cases of vCJD in France, which has the second highest number of cases of vCJD, has been estimated at 33. The modelling suggests that a large vCJD epidemic in France is very unlikely. The authors further suggest that as France was the recipient of 60% of the total British exports of bovine carcasses, their results should be reassuring for most countries worldwide [52].

From experimental studies it is known that scrapie and BSE induced in sheep can be transmitted by blood transfusion, and observational studies in humans confirm the transmission of vCJD in humans. Rodent study data suggest that the infectivity level via the intravenous route may be in the region of 10 infectious doses per mL (10 ID/mL), and prions are partitioned between plasma and leucocytes with 40 to 70 percent associated with leucocytes and negligible levels associated with red cells and platelets [53,54].

The United Kingdom, experiencing the greatest number of cases of vCJD, implemented a number of strategies to minimise the risk of transfusion transmission of prions [40]. These strategies were designed to

a) reduce exposure to donor plasma;

b) reduce exposure to donor leucocytes;
c) reduce the number of donor exposures;
d) defer previously transfused donors;
e) encourage appropriate transfusion practices; and
f) encourage use of alternatives to transfusions.

These strategies were achieved by non-use of UK plasma for fractionation and importing all plasma for fractionation from the USA, by importation of clinical fresh frozen plasma for younger transfusion recipients who had not been exposed to BSE, by universal leucodepletion of fresh blood products, by increasing the proportion of apheresis platelets, by deferral of previously transfused donors and by vigorous promotion of good transfusion practice.

Other countries adopted some of these measures according to the level of risk in their individual countries (Table 3).

Several countries adopted donor deferral strategies. For example, France deferred donors who had spent a cumulative period of one year or more in the UK between 1980 and 1996. Australia deferred donors who had spent a cumulative period of six months of more in the UK between 1 January 1980 and 31 December 1996, the USA deferred donors who had spent 3 months or more in the UK or who had resided in Europe for 5 years or longer since 1980. Japan deferred donors who had spent any time in the UK between 1980 and 1996, as well as those who had spent 6 months or more in the UK between 1997 and 2004. Several countries also deferred donors who had been transfused in the UK (and some also in Europe) between 1980 and the present time. The Food and Drug Administration issued draft guidelines in 2006 proposing the indefinite deferral of donors who have been transfused in France since 1980. Some countries also deferred donors who had been treated with European-derived bovine insulin.

The variety of measures adopted by individual countries to reduce the risk of transfusion transmitted vCJD were precautionary in nature and, in several countries (in the absence of sensitive and specific tests for screening potential donors), were based on risk modelling. In countries such as Australia, where up to 30 percent of the population had travelled to or resided in the UK between 1980 and 1996, the level of risk reduction had to be balanced with maintenance of the sufficiency of the blood supply. The loss of donors (5% of regular donors in Australia) also had to be balanced against the risk of a potential increase in other transfusion transmitted infections such as HIV, HCV and HBV, which have a higher prevalence in new compared with established repeat donors [55].

While most screening tests aim to detect PrP^{SC}, there is no reliable information on correlation of detection of PrP^{SC} with infectivity nor any certainty about the implications of a positive test for the donor [40]. It has been estimated that infectivity in blood might be four or even six orders of magnitude lower than in brain, with 1 ID/mL of blood obtained from scrapie-infected hamsters to be equivalent to 1 pg/mL of PrP^{SC}. While a multitude of techniques for detection of prions both in tissues and blood have been described, none has yet been licensed as a screening assay for human use. These tests include immunocapillary electrophoresis using a competitive inhibition, conformation dependant immunoassay using the binding differences of the 3F4 monoclonal antibody to PrP^{C} and PrP^{TSE}, a system for detecting multimers in plasma and tests using PrP^{TSE}.

Other assays such as the protein misfolding cyclic amplification (PMCA) are based on the principle that small amounts of PrP^{TSE} can convert excess amounts of PrP^{C} into PrP^{TSE} [56]. With repeated cycles of template based conversion and sonication to fragment the aggregated abnormal prion, PrP^{TSE} can be amplified to levels capable of detection in immunoassays. A variation of this assay using recombinant PrP as substrate and automated shaking instead of sonication is called the quaking induced conversion (QIC) assay.

Perhaps the most promising assay at the present time is the assay developed by Amorfix[4]. This so called epitope protection assay (EP-vCJD) uses peroxynitrite to selectively mask PrP^{C} epitopes. Aggregated PrP^{TSE} is protected, but when disaggregated these epitopes can be detected in a standard immunoassay.

Table 3. Matrix of Measures Taken to Prevent Transmission of vCJD by Transfusion

	FDA	American Red Cross	Canadian Blood Service	Hema-Quebec	Australia	New Zealand	United Kingdom
Donor Deferral							
UK							
≥ 1 year							
≥ 6 months					Yes	Yes	
≥ 3 months	Yes	Yes	Yes				
≥ 1 month				Yes			
France							
≥ 5 years	Yes	Yes					
≥ 6 months						Yes	
≥ 3 months			Yes	Yes			
Ireland							
≥ 6 months						Yes	
Europe							
≥ 5 years	Yes – SD plasma donors excepted	Yes	Yes				
≥ 6 months				Yes			
≥ 6 months US military bases	Yes	Yes					
Saudi Arabia							
≥ 6 months				Yes			
Transfusion							
UK							
Since 1980	Yes		Yes		Yes	Yes	
Any time		Yes					
France	Yes		Yes			Yes	
Ireland						Yes	
Western Europe			Yes	Yes			
Anywhere							Yes
Surgery in UK							
Plasma Fractionation							Import US plasma
Clinical FFP							Imported for neonates
Leucodepletion		Yes	Yes	Yes	Yes	Yes	Yes
Bovine Insulin	Yes	Yes	Yes[1]	Yes[1]	Yes	Yes[1]	

[4] Amorfix Life Science (Toronto, Canada)

Table 3. (Continued)

	Japan	Hong Kong	Singapore	France	Swiss Red Cross	Ireland
Donor Deferral						
UK						
≥ 1 year				Yes		Yes
≥ 6 months	Yes ('97-'04)		Yes		Yes	
≥ 3 months		Yes				
≥ 1 month	1 day ('80-'96)					
France						
≥ 5 years		Yes	Yes			
≥ 6 months	Yes					
≥ 3 months						
Ireland						
≥ 6 months	Yes					
Europe						
≥ 5 years	(Eastern '80-) (Aus,Gr,Swe,Den,Fin,Lux'80-'04)	Yes	Plasma only			
≥ 6 months	Western Eur/ Switzerland					
≥ 6 months US military bases		Yes				
Saudi Arabia						
≥ 6 months						
Transfusion						
UK						
Since 1980		Yes	Yes			
Any time						
France						
Ireland						
Western Europe						
Anywhere	Yes			Yes	Yes	Yes
Surgery in UK						Yes
Plasma Fractionation						
Clinical FFP						
Leucodepletion			Yes	Yes	Yes	Yes
Bovine Insulin		Yes	Yes[1]			

[1] Falls under category of insulin-dependent diabetes.

This assay has now been used to screen brain-spiked donor samples and has a high sensitivity. Further studies are proceeding to determine the true sensitivity and specificity of the assay.

One of the problems standing in the way of validation of candidate tests for vCJD in blood is the lack of appropriate vCJD positive plasma panels stored in a format suitable to assess potential screening assays. Spiked samples using brain and spleen homogenates are used, although doubts remain about the physical state of prions in such spiked samples and their relevance to natural infection. A second problem relates to the development of reliable confirmatory assays. It has been estimated that in the UK, which collects approximately 2.5 million donation a year and with a possible prevalence of 1 in 10,000 of subclinical vCJD, an assay with 99% specificity and sensitivity would result in approximately 25,000 false positive tests per year [57]. Such a high number of false positive tests in the absence of robust confirmatory tests would generate impossible donor management scenarios for transfusion services. Even a test with 99.5% specificity would produce 12,500 false reactive results in the first year of testing, and a specificity of 99.9% would still produce roughly 2,500 false reactives. Specificity becomes even more of a problem in those countries expected to have much lower rates of subclinical infection in blood donors such as Asia-Pacific countries. The ethical, legal social, medical and economic issues associated with the application of tests designed to screen the blood supply are addressed in a very comprehensive recent UK Department of Health report [58].

The UK is expected to lead the way in validation of a screening test when one becomes available, and it has been proposed that there should be a study of 50,000 blood donors using 5,000 USA plasma samples as a negative control panel. However, before such a study is undertaken it will be necessary for tiered preclinical studies, firstly by detection of blinded samples from dilutions of plasma pools spiked with infected brain and spleen homogenates, and if successful screening infected animal plasma samples and then available endogenously infected human plasma samples.

The issues relating to the potential contamination of the blood supply by vCJD in the Asia-Pacific region are different from those affecting Europe, with its proximity to the UK particularly and its extensive import, export and travel networks which may have facilitated spread of BSE before its significance as an infectious disease was realised.

Australia and New Zealand, for example, are considered to be BSE free and they are also scrapie free. Testing programs continue to assure freedom from BSE. Regulatory agencies in Australia have assured that products potentially contaminated by BSE are not imported into Australia. Furthermore, the National Health and Medical Research Council (NHMRC) established a Special Expert Committee on Transmissible Spongiform Encephalopathies (now called the TSE Advisory Committee) in 2002, and this committee has monitored all aspects of animal, food, medical, transfusion and transplantation issues arising from the BSE and vCJD epidemics. New Zealand has a similar committee with the same responsibilities (the TSE Steering Committee). Information about exposure to BSE in many non-European countries is not definitely known.

Although the extent of spread of subclinical infection is currently unknown, as described above, risk assessments suggest that the major risk to the blood supply in any individual country is related to the extent of residency of blood donors in the UK and, to a lesser extent, residency in other affected European countries (especially France) between 1980 and 1996. It has also been suggested that the major risk of exposure to BSE contaminated beef and bovine products in the UK was between 1988 and 1993. Deferral of donors who have lived in the UK for a cumulative arbitrary period in the risk years for BSE should reduce the risk of contamination of the blood supply, although other routes of infection such as contaminated neurosurgical, ophthalmological and endoscopic biopsy instruments as well as transplantation may pose additional risks if donors subject to these procedures are not deferred. Risk modelling shows that the added policy of deferral of blood donors who have been previously transfused in the UK (with or without the addition of deferral for previous transfusion in France) at any time since 1980 should further limit the risk of transmission by blood transfusion.

In the absence of a sensitive screening test, an alternative approach has been the development of filters capable of removing prions from blood. Such prion filtration steps have been developed for plasma pools during the manufacture of fractionated products. Several companies are now in the process of developing prion removal filters for whole blood and blood components.

Pall[5] has developed a polyester fibre filter (Leucotrap Affinity Reduction Filter) whose surface binds prions in leucodepleted red cells. One study used human red cells spiked with brain homogenate from scrapie-infected hamsters with the removal of 3.7 log ID/mL by Bioassay [59]. The second study used endogenously infected hamster blood during the clinical phase of the disease. Six of 187 animals who received non-filtered red cells injected into their brain developed clinical symptoms caused by PrP^{SC}, but one recipient of filtered red cells also became infected. The filter has been redesigned as a combined leucodepletion and prion filter and is undergoing further evaluation.

MacoPharma[6] have also developed a filter, the PA-Capt filter which incorporates a ligand marketed by PRDT[7]. The filter material binds with high affinity abnormal prions from both classical and variant CJD and from scapie-infected hamster brain. Human red cells spiked with scrapie-infected brain homogenate and filtered removed infectivity below the level of detection by western blot and by 4 log ID/mL in Bioassay. Intracerebral inoculation of scrapie-infected brain-spiked prion-filtered red cells into 100 hamsters showed a reduction of 2.8 ID/mL of blood infectivity with no infected hamsters up to 18 months post inoculation.

Asahi Kasei[8] has also developed a combined leucoreduction prion reduction filter by modification of the filter surface with a polymer. Preliminary results show a reduction of prion proteins by more than 3.5 logs with substantial reduction of leucocytes.

Currently, although early results are indicative [60], the results of definitive clinical evaluation studies such as measurement of haemolysis of red cells as well as effects on plasma proteins (including coagulation factors and complement proteins) during the filtration process when applied to human blood donations are awaited.

Pathogen inactivation, which has been shown to be effective against a wide variety of infectious agents such as bacteria, viruses and parasites, is not effective against prions.

Given the many uncertainties still surrounding prion disease in general and vCJD in particular, the issues associated with the prevention of transfusion transmitted vCJD are complex. Given the experimental evidence in animal models and the human cases of putative transfusion transmission by non-leucodepleted red cells and more recently by a fractionated plasma product, concern for the safety of the blood supply is warranted. Although there has been only one documented case in the Asia-Pacific region to date, the long incubation period of the disease, the potential for subclinical and preclinical infections (particularly in non methionine homozygous individuals) and the significant implications for public health, the precautionary approach taken by many countries is essential.

The prevalence of vCJD in individual countries may depend on a number of factors. These include:

- the importation of infected cattle and beef products from the UK and to a lesser extent Europe in the years before BSE was recognised and controlled;

---

[5] Pall Corporation (East Hills NY, USA)
[6] MacoPharma (Tourcoing, France)
[7] Pathogen Removal and Diagnostic Technology (Falls Church VA, USA)
[8] Asahi Kasei Medical (Oita, Japan)

- the proportion of the population who may have been exposed during travel to or residence in UK and other risk countries;
- the number of imported blood components and blood products from BSE risk countries; and
- the proportion of the population who might have been transfused in the UK or other at-risk European countries.

For blood transfusion services a risk assessment based on the available information on the potential exposure of blood donors to prions is the best approach to safeguard the blood supply. Risk reduction measures can then be based on improving safety balanced against the sufficiency of the blood supply in each country. In the absence of sensitive and specific screening tests, donor deferral strategies are the easiest of a number of measures to institute provided sufficiency is not threatened and safety is not further compromised by the recruitment of new replacement donors who may be at higher risk of other infectious diseases.

Leucodepletion is also a risk reduction step, but comes at considerable cost despite the additional benefits unrelated to reduction of prions. Prion filters (should validation trials show that there are no untoward effects on red cells, platelets or plasma proteins) may be applicable in some countries, but again will come at considerable cost.

Finally, the availability of sensitive and specific screening tests will offer a more definitive approach to eliminating the transfusion risk. Screening tests however will be difficult to institute without a gold standard confirmatory test. The ethical, legal, social and economic costs will be considerable, and it is likely that countries in the Asia -Pacific region will not implement testing procedures until many of these complex issues have been addressed in the UK and France, which have the greatest burden of disease at the present time.

It is recognised that in many countries the problems of other infectious disease (eg malaria and dengue) may be of much greater significance to the safety of the blood supply than vCJD at the present time, and currently much more significant in the cost benefit equation. Nevertheless, sharing of expertise and cooperation in the region, for example by involvement in collaborative studies, may help all our Asia-Pacific countries to weave a path through the complexities of transfusion-transmitted prion disease and to maximise the safety of the blood supply in our region.

The Future

Technology advances continue to provide the potential to refine testing practices and reduce the overall risk of TTI. For example, new automated NAT systems have evolved from first generation 'semi-automated'systems [61]. These have expanded the existing capacity to screen for HIV and HCV RNA to include Hepatitis B DNA in a 'triplex' assay format. As well as providing the mechanism to further reduce the risk of transfusion transmitted HBV particularly in high prevalence populations, they offer improved process control (virtually eliminating 'human' errors) and improved cost effectiveness. A number of countries have implemented these triplex assays with the aim of reducing the risk of window period HBV infection and/or occult HBV infection [62].

Microarray technology offers perhaps the most promising 'next generation' blood testing platform. Petrik and co-workers describe microarrays as 'miniaturised solid phase assays of high multiplexing power' [63]. These have the potential to screen for multiple agents on a single tailored 'chip' although currently the hurdle of combining protein and nucleic acid targets is an elusive goal. Developed to their full potential, microarrays could revolutionise blood screening offering rapid and inexpensive tailored testing for infectious disease markers (both protein and nucleic acid) in parallel with blood grouping antigens.

Pathogen reduction methods have been used widely in the manufacture of pooled plasma derived proteins reducing the risk of infection from these products to near zero [64]. Physicochemical pathogen reduction techniques for individual blood components have been under development for some time and recent progress particularly with plasma and platelets has led to increasing application of the these technologies [65]. The key advantage of these techniques is their potential to reduce or eliminate the risk of known pathogens as well as those that might emerge in the future. Despite the immense potential there are several limitations with the currently available methods that have to date precluded any from being implemented in either Australia or North America. First, no single method can be applied to all blood components. Second, existing 'safety' levels in voluntary donors are very high as a result of current risk reduction strategies (e.g. donor selection, testing and surveillance for known/emerging pathogens). Third, some methods are unable to inactivate certain pathogens including prions, spores and non enveloped viruses. Fourth, there are continuing concerns over the toxicity of residual chemical agents used in some methods. Finally, there is a perception that available techniques may well lack cost effectiveness when compared with other available interventions to address non infectious transfusion threats [66]. Despite these challenges the potential to remove all infectious agents with a single processing step remains a compelling driver to continue development of these methods [33]. Undoubtedly, blood services worldwide will continue to monitor the progress of pathogen reduction techniques with keen interest.

Infectious diseases in the context of today's 'global village' know no boundaries. The frequency and rapidity of international travel provide an efficient transport mechanism for existing, and perhaps more significantly novel agents. This new paradigm was well demonstrated during the 2002 SARS outbreak with a novel virus rapidly spreading from its epicenter in China to Hong Kong, Singapore and to Canada and subsequently threatening the remainder of the globe [1]. The lessons learned during the SARS outbreak have been further honed and are being applied to the current threat of influenza pandemic posed by the epizootic avian influenza A (H5N1) virus. These include the need for:

- transparent and timely outbreak reporting;
- unfettered sharing of relevant clinical and scientific data including access to genetic material;
- regular international conferences/forums to address emerging disease threats; and
- comprehensive national and international response plans for significant threats such as HIV/AIDS, and pandemic influenza.

By acting 'globally' the likelihood of success in mitigating the myriad of infectious risks is undoubtedly optimised but history reveals that man is seldom a match for nature!

Conclusion

Despite the obvious potential for blood transfusion to act as an efficient vehicle for transmitting viruses, current microbial safety interventions have proven to be extremely effective in preventing infection with recognised viruses. As risks from new agents are identified (usually after transmission is demonstrated), where available, interventions may be implemented if justified by the level of risk. If it is considered necessary to prevent such risks prospectively (rather than retrospectively) then 'catch-all' interventions such as pathogen reduction may have to be considered. Finally, the risk of emergence of transfusion transmissible infectious diseases emphasises the need for countries to work together to help each other maintain their blood supplies during epidemics and pandemics. This is particularly important should a major infectious disease pandemic occur in different countries at different times.

References

[1] Vijayanand P, Wilkins E, Woodhead M. Severe acute respiratory syndrome (SARS): a review. *Clin Med* 2004;4: 152-60.

[2] Will RG, Ironside JW, Zeidler M, *et al.* A new variant of Creutzfeldt-Jakob disease in the UK. *Lancet* 1996;347: 921-5.

[3] Dodd R. Other emerging viral pathogens. *ISBT Science Series* 2006;1: 257-62.

[4] Heneine W, Kuehnert MJ. Preserving blood safety against emerging retroviruses. *Transfusion* 2006;46: 1276-8.

[5] Dodd RY, Leiby DA. Emerging Infectious Threats to the Blood Supply *Annu. Rev. Med.* 2004;55: 191-207.

[6] Kleinman S. West Nile virus and transfusion safety in North America: response to an emerging pathogen. *ISBT Science Series* 2006;1: 251-6.

[7] Seed CR, Kiely P, Keller AJ. Residual risk of transfusion transmitted human immunodeficiency virus, hepatitis B virus, hepatitis C virus and human T lymphotrophic virus. *Intern Med J* 2005;35: 592-8.

[8] Bihl F, Castelli D, Marincola F, *et al.* Transfusion-transmitted infections. *Journal of Translational Medicine* 2007;5: 1-11.

[9] Polizzotto MN, E.M. W, Ingham H, Keller AJ. Reducing the risk of transfusion-transmissible viral infection through blood donor selection: the Australian experience 2000 through 2006. *Transfusion* 2008;48: 55-63.

[10] Mison L, Seed CR, Margaritis AR, Hyland C. Nucleic acid technology screening of Australian blood donors for hepatitis C and human immunodeficiency virus-1 RNA: comparison of two high-throughput testing strategies. *Vox Sang* 2003;84: 11-9.

[11] Epstein JS. Insights on donor screening for West Nile virus. *Transfusio*n 2005;45: 460-2.

[12] Zou S. Potential impact of pandemic influenza on blood safety and availability. *Transfus Med Rev* 2006;20: 181-9.

[13] Alter HJ. Emerging,re-emerging and submerging infectious threats to the blood supply (abstract). *Vox sanguinis* 2004;87 (Supplement 2): 56.

[14]Lindsay M, Mackenzie JS. Vector-borne viral diseases and climate change in the Australasian region:Major concerns and the public health response. In: Curson P, ed. *Climate change and human health in the Asia-Pacific region: Blackwell-Synergy*, 1998.

[15]Chuang VW, Wong TY, Leung YH, *et al.* Review of dengue fever cases in Hong Kong during 1998 to 2005. *Hong Kong Med J* 2008;14: 170-7.

[16]Tambyah PA, Koay ES, Poon ML, *et al.* Dengue hemorrhagic fever transmitted by blood transfusion. *N Engl J Med* 2008;359: 1526-7.

[17]Nash D, Mostashari F, Fine A, *et al.* The outbreak of West Nile virus infection in the New York City area in 1999. *New Engl J Med* 2001;344: 1807-14.

[18]Busch MP, Wright DJ, Custer B, *et al.* West Nile virus infections projected from blood donor screening data, United States, 2003. *Emerg Infect Dis* 2006;12: 395-402.

[19]Mackenzie JS, Smith DW, Hall RA. West Nile Virus: is there a message for Australia? *Med J Aust* 2003;178: 5-6.

[20]Ligon BL. Dengue fever and dengue hemorrhagic fever: a review of the history, transmission, treatment, and prevention. *Semin Pediatr Infect Dis* 2005;16: 60-5.

[21]Russell RC, Dwyer DE. Arboviruses associated with human disease in Australia. *Microbes and Infection* 2000;14: 1693-704.

[22]Charrel RN, de Lamballerie X, Raoult D. Chikungunya outbreaks - The Globalization of vectorborne diseases. *New Engl J Med* 2007;356: 769-71.

[23]Druce JD, Johnson DF, Tran T, *et al.* Chikungunya virus infection in a traveler to Australia (letter). *Emerg Infect Dis* 2007;13: 509-10.

[24]Johnson DF, Druce JD, Chapman S, *et al.* Chikungunya virus infection in travellers to Australia. *Med J Aust* 2008;188: 41-3.

[25]Liumbuno G, Catalano L, Pupella S, *et al.* The Chikungunya epidemic in Italy and its impact on the blood supply (abstract). *Transfusion* 2008;48 (Supplement): 24A.

[26]Leroy EM, Baisze S, Volchkov VE, *et al.* Human asymptomatic Ebola infection and strong inflammatory response. *Lancet* 2000;355: 2178-9.

[27]Eaton BT, Mackenzie JS, Wang LF. Henipaviruses. In: Knipe DM, Howley, P.M., ed. *Fields Virology*. Philidelphia: Wolters Kluwer: Lippincott, Williams & Wilkins, 2007:1587-600.

[28]Guertler LG. Virus safety of human blood, plasma and derived products. *Thrombosis Research* 2002;107: S39-S45.

[29]Palacios G, Druce JD, Tran T, *et al.* A new arenavirus in a cluster of fatal transplant-associated diseases. *New Engl J Med* 2008;358: 1-8.

[30]Likos AM, Kelvin DJ, Cameron CM, *et al.* Influenza viremia and the potential for blood-borne transmission. *Transfusion* 2007;47: 1080-8.

[31]Nishizawa T, Okamoto H, Konishi K, *et al.* A novel DNA virus (TTV) associated with elevated transaminase levels in posttransfusion hepatitis of unknown etiology. *Biochem Biophys Res Commun* 1997;241: 92-7.

[32]Tanaka Y, Primi D, Wang RY, *et al.* Genomic and molecular evolutionary analysis of a newly identified infectious agent (SEN virus) and its relationship to the TT virus family. *J Infect Dis* 2001;183: 359-67.

[33]Alter HJ, Stramer SL, Dodd RY. Emerging infectious diseases that threaten the blood supply. *Semin Hematol* 2007;44: 32-41.

[34]Australian Government Department of Health and Ageing. *National Notifiable Diseases Network Surveillance System [monograph on the internet]*. Canberra; 2007. Available from: http://www.health.gov.au/cda

[35]Communicable Disease Australia. *Communicable Diseases Network of Australia [monograph on the internet]*. Canberra; 2007. Available from: www.health.gov.au/cda

[36]Kitchen AD, Barbara JA. Which agents threaten blood safety in the future? *Baillieres Best Pract Res Clin Haematol* 2000;13: 601-14.

[37]Seed C, Kiely P, Hyland C, Keller AJ. Estimating the risk of dengue transmission by blood transfusion during a 2004 Australian outbreak (abstract). *Transfusion* 2008;48: 25A.

[38]Will RG, Ironside JW, Zeidler M, Cousens SN, Estibeiro K, Alperovitch A, Poser S, Pocchiari M, Hofman A, Smith PG. A new variant of Creutzfeldt-Jakob disease in the UK. *Lancet* 1996; 347(9006): 921-925.

[39]Bruce ME, Will RG, Ironside JW, McConnell I, Drummond D, Suttie A, McCardle L, Chree A, Hope J, Birkett C, Cousens S, Fraser H, Bostock CJ. Transmissions to mice indicate that 'new variant' CJD is caused by the BSE agent. *Nature* 1997; 389(6650): 498-501.

[40]Coste J, Prowse C, Eglin R, Fang C for the Subgroup on TSE. A report on transmissible spongiform encephalopathies and transfusion safety. *Vox Sang* 2009; 96(4):284-291.

[41]Gregori L, Rohwer RG. Characterization of scrapie-infected and normal hamster blood as an experimental model for TSE-infected human blood. *Dev Biol (Basel)* 2007; 127: 123-133.

[42]Hunter N, Foster J, Chong A, McCutcheon S, Parnham D, Eaton S, Mackenzie C, Houston F. Transmission of prion diseases by blood transfusion. *J Gen Virol* 2002; 83(Pt 11): 2897-2905.

[43]Houston F, McCutcheon S, Goldman W, Chong A, Foster J, Sisó S, González L, Jeffrey M, Hunter N. Prion diseases are efficiently transmitted by blood transfusion in sheep. *Blood* 2008; 112(2): 4739-4745.

[44]European and Allied Countries Collaborative Study Group of vCJD. CJD statistics 2009. http://www.eurocjd.ed.ac.uk/vcjdworldeuro.htm

[45]Lefrère JJ, Hewitt P. From mad cows to sensible blood transfusion: the risk of prion transmission by labile blood components in the United Kingdom and in France. *Transfusion* 2009; 49(4): 797-812.

[46]Hewitt PE, Llewelyn CA, Mackenzie J, Will RG. Creutzfeldt-Jakob disease and blood transfusion: results of the UK Transfusion Medicine Epidemiological Review study. *Vox Sang* 2006; 91(3): 221-230.

[47]Bennett P, Ball J. vCJD risk assessment calculations for a patient with multiple routes of exposure.http://www.dh.gov.uk/en/Publicationsandstatistics/Publications/PublicationsPolicyAndGuidance/DH_100357.

[48]Hilton DA, Ghani AC, Conyers L, Edwards P, McCardle L, Ritchie D, Penney M, Hegazy D, Ironside JW. Prevalence of lymphoreticular prion protein accumulation in UK tissue samples. *J Pathol* 2004; 203(3): 733-739.

[49]Peden AH, Head MW, Ritchie DL, Bell JE, Ironside JW. Preclinical vCJD after blood transfusion in a PRNP codon 129 heterozygous patient. *Lancet* 2004; 364(9433): 527-529.

[50]Clewley JP, Kelly CM, Andrews N, Vogliqi K, Mallison G, Hilton DA, Ironside JW, Edwards P, McCardle LM, Ritchie DL, Dabaghian R, Ambrose HE, Gill ON. Prevalence of disease related prion protein in anonymous tonsil specimens in Britain: cross sectional opportunistic survey. *BMJ* 2009; 338: b1442.

[51]Watts S. Fears raised over new vCJD wave. BBC Online 17 Dec 2008. http://news.bbc.co.uk/1/hi/health/7788627.stm.

[52]Chadeau-Hyam M, Alpérovitch A. Risk of variant Creutzfeldt-Jakob disease in France. *Int J Epidemiol* 2005; 34(1): 46-52.

[53]Holada K, Vostal JG, Theisen PW, MacAuley C, Gregory L, Rohwer RG. Scrapie infectivity in hamster blood is not associated with platelets. *J Virol* 2002; 76(9): 4649-4650.

[54]Dobra SA, Bennett PG. vCJD and blood transfusion: risk assessment in the United Kingdom. *Transfus Clin Biol* 2006; 13(5): 307-316.

[55]Correll PK, Law MG, Seed CR, Gust A, Buhring M, Dax EM, Keller AJ, Kaldor JN. Variant Creutzfeldt-Jakob disease in Australian blood donors: estimation of risk and the impact of deferral strategies. *Vox Sanguinis* 2001; 81: 6-11.

[56]Saborio GP, Permanne B, Soto C. Sensitive detection of pathological prion protein by cyclic amplification of protein misfolding. *Nature* 2001; 411(6839): 810-813.

[57]Turner M. Transfusion safety with regards to prions: ethical, legal and social considerations. *Transfus Clin Biol* 2006; 13(5): 317-319.

[58]Bennett P, Dobra S Mapping out the consequences of screening blood donations for PrP^{SC} www.dh.gov.uk/en/Publicationsandstatistics/Publications/PublicationsPolicyAndGuidance/DH 094804.

[59]Sowemino-Coker SO, Pesci S, Andrade F, Kim A, Kascsak RB, Kascsak RJ, Meeker C, Carp R. Pall Leucotrap affinity prion-reduction filter removes exogenous infectious prions and endogenous infectivity from red cell concentrates. *Vox Sang* 2006; 90(4): 265-275.

[60]Murphy CV, Eakins E, Fagan J, Croxon H, Murphy WG. *In vitro* assessment of red-cell concentrates in SAG-M filtered through the MacoPharma™ P-CAPT prion-reduction filter. *Transfus Med* 2009; 19(3): 109-116.

[61]Margaritis AR, Brown SM, Seed CR, *et al.* Comparison of two automated nucleic acid testing systems for simultaneous detection of human immunodeficiency virus and hepatitis C virus RNA and hepatitis B virus DNA. *Transfusion* 2007;47: 1783-93.

[62]Lelie N, Heaton A. Hepatitis B - A review of the role of NAT in enhancing blood safety. *J of Clin Virol* 2006;36 (supplement 1): S1-S2.

[63]Petrik J, de Haas M, Denomme G, *et al.* Small world - Advance of microarrays: Current status and future trends. *Transfus Aph Sci* 2007;36: 201-6.

[64]Burnouf T, Radosevich M. Reducing the risk of infection from plasma products: specific preventative strategies. *Blood Rev* 2000;14: 94-110.

[65]Bryant BJ, Klein H. Pathogen Inactivation - The definitive safeguard for the blood supply. *Arch Pathol Lab Med* 2007;131: 719-33.

[66]Klein H, Anderson D, M-J. B, *et al.* Pathogen inactivation: making decisions about new technologies - preliminary report of a consensus conference. *Vox Sang* 2007;93: 179-82.

INDEX

A

B

C

F

G

H

M

N

O

P

Q

R

S

T

U

V

W

Y